Recipe
for a
Healthy
Brain

This is a work of nonfiction. The events and conversations in this book have been set down to the best of the author's ability, although some names and details may have been changed to protect the privacy of individuals. Every effort has been made to trace or contact all copyright holders. The publishers will be pleased to make good any omissions or rectify any mistakes brought to their attention at the earliest opportunity.

Printed in Australia

Cover design by Shawline Publishing Group Pty Ltd

Images in this book are the copyright of Shawline Publishing Group Pty Ltd

Illustrations within this book are the copyright of Shawline Publishing Group Pty Ltd

First Printing: May 2022

Shawline Publishing Group Pty Ltd
www.shawlinepublishing.com.au

Paperback ISBN- 9781922701312

Ebook ISBN- 9781922701343

A catalogue record for this book is available from the National Library of Australia

Recipe for a Healthy Brain

DR ROY HARDMAN &
DR MELISSA FORMICA

Acknowledgments:

My sincerest appreciation goes out to Dr Roy Hardman for inviting me to partake in this exciting journey with him.

I sincerely want to thank my co-author Dr Melissa Formica for her magnificent support and enthusiastic approach to this very important topic.

Index:

Forward:

This publication is based on the science of published data, not hear-say, popular (pop) psychology or pop-science of unqualified opinions.

If you are seriously interested in ways to avoid venturing towards age-related onset of dementia and want to live a long and healthy life and reduce the risk of dementia, then this is the text for you.

There are no half-backed ideas, popular diets, or fads expressed in this publication; only well documented scientific assessment of the facts.

Profile of Authors:

Dr Roy J Hardman

Roy gained his PhD from the Faculty of Health Science at Swinburne University of Technology within the Centre for Human Psychopharmacology Melbourne, Australia. Roy's research 'Effects of adherence to a Mediterranean style diet and healthy lifestyle on cognitive functioning in independently living older individuals' The 'LIILAC' study (Lifestyle Intervention, Independently living Aged Care) is a 2x2 factorial design, random control pilot trial which has been published widely in the academic press. Roy has also been a co-author with other research papers and was part of the research team in Australia for The Med Walk trial, an NHMRC funded trial. Roy and his college Dr Melissa Formica also collaborated writing the chapter on 'Mediterranean Diet and Cognition' as part of the 2nd edition Mediterranean textbook from Kings College Cambridge in 2020 and Advances in Health and Disease Vol 35 in the USA in 2021. Together Roy and Melisa have published "My Brain is My Best Friend"; a children's book focused on how to eat for a healthy brain. There are three more children's books in the works over the next couple of years. Roy also has a research background in Biochemistry and Drug Metabolism with the combination of Wellness Research together with over 30 years of working within the health care industry in Australia and worldwide.

Dr Melissa Formica

Melissa completed an Honours degree in Psychology and then went on to complete her PhD with an Australian Postgraduate Award scholarship at Deakin University. Melissa has published her work investigating the effects of diet and exercise on maintaining cognitive function in older adults and has also co-published the chapter on 'Mediterranean Diet and Cognition' as part of the 2nd edition Mediterranean textbook from Kings College Cambridge in 2020. Melissa currently works as a Research Fellow at Barwon Health, Geelong. Her main research interests include the impact of lifestyle factors on maintaining cognitive function into old age and avoiding cognitive decline following surgery. Melissa has also completed her Master's degree and is training to become registered as a general psychologist.

CHAPTER 1:

How does our Brain Age Physically?

As with every other organ in the body, our brain will age as we get older. The impact of this ageing process on an individual's brain depends on the amount of nurturance with regard to development and 'exercise' over their lifetime (Yankner, Lu, & Loerch, 2008), as brain ageing is considered the progressive and gradual accumulation of potential detrimental changes in brain cellular structure and function (Mattson, Chan, & Duan, 2002). This means that changes build up over the course of our lifetime and are dependent on many factors such as the things we eat, how often we exercise and how stressful our lives are. Given everyone's lives are different, these changes do not occur to the same extent in every person or brain region (Fratiglioni, Mangialasche, & Qiu, 2010; Peters, 2006).

Age-related changes occur at multiple levels. This includes:

- The neural and cellular level
- The regional level

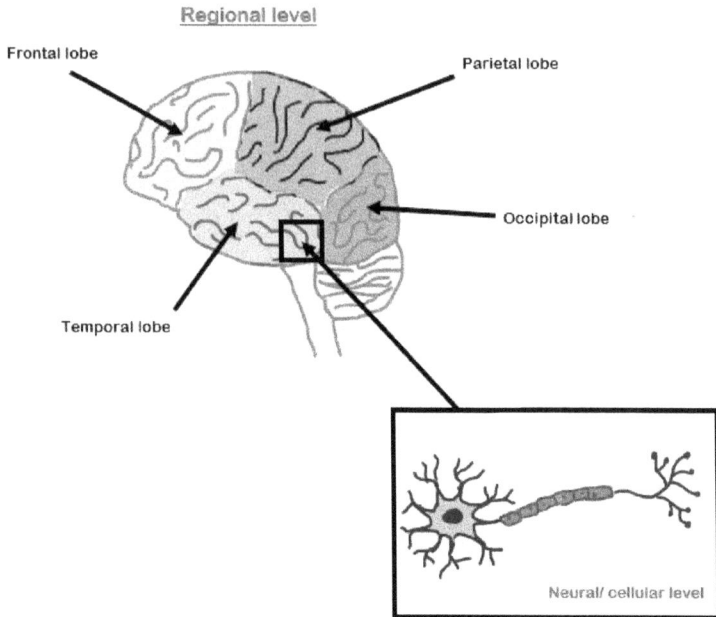

It is important to have a basic understanding of the role of each of these before we can understand how we can target interventions to avoid detrimental impacts during our lifetime.

The 'neural' level

The **neural level** is the cell level of the brain that forms the building blocks for development and functionality. The brain responds to environmental demands by producing new proteins to preserve the integrity of the brain, referred to as neurons. This means that changes to **neurons** can occur quite frequently, even across the course of a day.

Neurons are the key to communication between different regions in the brain. Their job is to receive information from our surroundings and to transport commands to different parts of our body to react to that information. This communication is facilitated by small molecules, referred to as **neurotransmitters**. The role of the neurotransmitters is to regulate adult neural development and cell growth, differentiate between the cells, and transmit messages across the gaps between nerve cells (synaptic transmission) (Behar, Schaffner, Scott, O'Connell, & Barker, 1998).

Sometimes, these neurons can become damaged due to a number of factors, including inflammation within cells, oxidative stress, and low energy levels at the cellular level (metabolic stress). Changes which result in the loss of neurons or neuronal organisation is referred to as **neurodegenerative** and impacts the brain in a negative fashion. Sometimes, these changes can occur concurrently, which is referred to as **cascades**. Consider a waterfall which becomes larger when more water is moving. The more changes occurring at once in the brain, the larger the area of damage, leading to **cognitive decline** (Mattson et al., 2002).

Neuronal damage builds up over time. It is perceived as age-related frailty, disability and disease (Kirkwood 2008). However, the brain can produce new neurons in response to stress factors it has been exposed to through a process called **neurogenesis**, bringing the brain back into balance. The extent to which your brain can create new neurons to balance damage will determine how severely your abilities are impacted. This response is referred to as being **neuroprotective**. It may be improved through changes in lifestyle factors such as diet and behavioural modifications.

The brain also has other compensatory mechanisms which allow it to continue functioning despite damages. One such compensatory mechanism is **dendritic sprouting.** This allows the ends of neurons to spread and make new connections with other nerve cells. These new connections allow the brain to maintain **cognitive reserve** with regard to functioning.

The cognitive reserve of an individual relates to how their brain is able to cope with neural damage by utilising compensatory mechanisms (Colombo, Antonietti, & Daneau, 2018). As such, it has been proposed that an individual with a higher cognitive reserve may be able to cope better with neural damage than an individual with a lower cognitive reserve (Colombo et al., 2018; Nilsson & Lovden, 2018). We will talk about ways to boost your cognitive reserve in later chapters.

The changes in the number and organisation of neurons that occur throughout the ageing process cannot be observed easily as they often include small and subtle changes. Often these changes require imaging methods to observe them ('Global Nutrition,' 2018; Park & Reuter-Lorenz, 2009). For instance, it has been demonstrated that gradual neuronal loss occurs in many important brain regions, including the neocortex (layers covering the brain responsible for higher-order functions such as motor commands, sensory perception and language), the hippocampus (the 'memory centre' of the brain) and disconnection between brain regions, particularly involving the prefrontal cortex (grey matter at the front of your brain responsible for higher-order functions) (Burke & Barnes, 2006; Yankner et al., 2008).

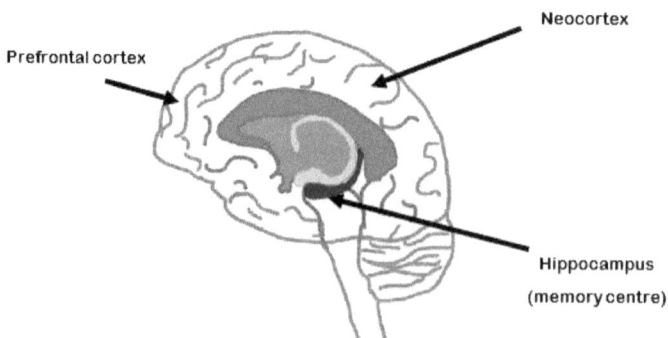

Neocortex

Prefrontal cortex

Hippocampus
(memory centre)

From a physical perspective, these small age-related changes add up over time and can be eventually identified by an overall reduction in brain volume and weight (Anderson, Åberg, Nilsson, & Eriksson, 2002). For example, it is predicted that brain volume decreases at a rate of 5% per decade after the age of 40 years and that this accelerates after 70 years of age (Peters, 2006).

White matter and grey matter are often known as the main 'substance' which makes up the brain. However, each has distinct functions which can be affected by ageing. White matter is constructed of what is referred to as **axon tracts.** Axon tracts are nerve tracts which are a bundle of nerve fibres not too dissimilar to what you see when cutting an electoral power cord and see the wires within. These tracts transmit the electrical signals within the brain cells. The fibre bundles are wrapped in a fatty layer called **myelin** which is made up of protein and fatty substances insulating the axons like the plastic or cotton on a power cord. This allows the fibres to conduct signals quickly and effectively. The type of fat in myelin makes it look white, so myelin-dense white matter takes on a white colour.

Grey matter, on the other hand, is a dense layer of neuron cell bodies and non-neuron brain cells called **glial cells**. The glial cells are also referred to as supporting cells of the nervous system. These cells have four main functions:

- they surround neurons and hold them in place
- they supply nutrients and oxygen to neurons
- they insulate one neuron from another and
- they destroy and remove the biological material of dead neurons

As glial cells are not surrounded by white myelin, they are a grey colour.

Long-term damage related to ageing at a neural level can therefore lead to cortical thinning (a reduction in the thickness of the brain's cortex), changes in grey and white matter and changes in the way that communication happens within and between different brain regions (Park and Reuter-Lorenz, 2009; Huizinga et al., 2018; Scheller et al., 2018). Specifically, a popular explanation regarding these changes is referred to as **The Retrogenesis Hypothesis.** This theory is often discussed regarding dementia and Alzheimer's disease (Reisberg et al., 1999). This theory suggests that damage to the axon fibres in our neurons is due to a substance called **amyloid**. Amyloid isn't normally found in the body- instead, it is produced by different proteins. Amyloid causes damage to the white matter resulting in a reduction in information transmission across brain regions that mediate higher cognitive function. This reduction results in what is referred to as the **Neuropsychological Syndrome.** This condition is characterized by behavioural and cognitive changes or, ultimately, a change in the relationship between one's brain and behaviour. This is considered to be one cause of Alzheimer's Disease.

How do we fuel our brains?

Given that the brain undergoes so many changes throughout the lifespan and even daily, it is not surprising that the brain requires a lot of energy. In fact, it is estimated that the brain consumes up to 20% of the total energy consumed by one's body.

Emerging literature suggests that the brain has different energy demands throughout an individual's life. For instance, babies and children require more energy than older adults as their bodies are growing and developing. This energy comes from the food that we eat. Therefore, changes in nutritional requirements are of great importance to accommodate changes in energy requirements across various periods of development (Coutre & Schmitt, 2008). As such, it is critical to understand the impacts of a poor versus optimal diet with respect to what may lead to a healthy brain and what drives transient cognitive performance.

It has been demonstrated that reduced energy and/or essential nutrient supply during the first stages of life can profoundly impact the brain's structural and functional development. Although in some cases, the brain's growth may proceed normally in the context of overall inadequate nutrition, the brain's structure may be altered if specific essential nutrients are absent (Uauy & Dangour, 2006). Specifically, it has been demonstrated that a foetus is dependent on maternal nutrients such as long-chain essential fatty acids, particularly n-3 long-chain polyunsaturated fatty acids.

Long-chain polyunsaturated fatty acids are dietary compounds found in fish. These are important for development as they play a role in neuronal growth, vision as well as psychomotor development, to name a few (Uauy, 2006). It has been suggested that at least a 0.3 g/day increment in dietary long-chain polyunsaturated fatty acids (approximately 1 serving/week of fatty fish intake) is required for adults (Chen, Yang, Eggersdorfer, Zhang, & Qin, 2016).

To have enough energy for the human brain to function, it is important to obtain the B-complex vitamins, including B1-thiamine, B2-riboflavin, B3-niacin, B5-pantothenate, B6-biotin, folate and B12-cobalamin, which produce neurotransmitter regulators. Published data suggests that there is a protective effect associated with B vitamins, particularly B12, B6 and folate (B9), with respect to cognitive function (Kennedy, 2016; Ordovas, 2008). Given their role in neurotransmitter regulation, the B-vitamins may affect energy, brain function and modulation of mood (Gesch, Hammond, Hampson, Eves, & Crowder, 2002). For instance, feelings of happiness and survival mechanisms such as fight-or-flight response may be attributed to the B vitamins, given their role in producing neurotransmitters such as serotonin, epinephrine, norepinephrine and gamma-aminobutyric acid (GABA) (Fernandes et al., 2008; Kennedy et al., 2016; Ordovas, 2008). It has also been found that Vitamin B6 is important for biochemical reactions which occur in the body. This is important not only in the brain but many organs such as the heart, kidneys, lungs and liver.

Vitamin E, beta-carotene and flavonoids, which are found in fruit and vegetables, may also have a protective effect against 'rusty brain' due to antioxidants. Like when iron combines with oxygen (oxidises) to form iron oxide or rust, a loss of electrons within the cell (oxidation) can occur within the brain. It is therefore thought that foods rich in antioxidants can reduce oxidative damage to the brain by enhancing the antioxidant defences (Van Dyk & Sano, 2007).

In addition to antioxidants, research has also suggested that plant polyphenols (a natural organic chemical) contained in fruits and vegetables interact with ageing neurons in the brain, increasing the neuron's capacity to maintain effective and proper functioning during the ageing process (Fernando Gomez-Pinilla, 2008).

Taken together, the evidence relating to the importance of a healthy diet for a healthy brain has led many researchers to suggest that a diet rich in B-vitamins, antioxidants and omega-3 essential fatty acids are required for a cognitively healthy brain during ageing (Van Dyk & Sano, 2007).

Although a lot of research has looked at the impact of single nutrients on the brain, the fact of the matter is that we do not simply consume individual nutrients; rather, we tend to adhere to a particular pattern with regards to the foods we eat. As such, emerging research is beginning to look at the effect of overall dietary habits over a lifetime on cognitive function ('Global Nutrition,' 2018). We will provide an overview of the evidence for the effects of different dietary patterns on cognitive function in Chapter 6.

Now that you have a basic understanding of how the brain works, the different areas of the brain and how the brain is typically affected during ageing, you will be able to build an understanding of the information provided in the following chapters regarding how various interventions work to prevent cognitive decline. You will be able to use this knowledge to decide what areas of your cognition you may be worried about, which will allow you to target your lifestyle modifications accordingly.

CHAPTER 2:

How does our Brain Age Cognitively?

So far, we have provided an overview of what the brain is and how it functions. Now that you have an understanding of the physical changes which occur in the brain during ageing, we will now consider cognitive changes. **Cognition** refers to any mental action or process of obtaining knowledge and understanding through thought, experience, and the senses.

Changes in cognitive abilities

Unsurprisingly, brain volume loss, which occurs in various regions of the brain associated with 'normal' ageing, has implications for many cognitive processes, including slowing. As such, it has been estimated that 40% of men and 46% of women over the age of 50 will experience some form of functional limitation (Jagger, Gillies, Moscone, & Team, 2008; Sourdet, Rouge-Bugat, Vellas, & Forette, 2012).

Like structural changes, it is important to note that the changes in the brain with respect to cognition is not necessarily the same between individuals (Christensen, 2003). When considering the cognitive abilities of an individual, it is essential to understand the three major classifications of abilities:

- crystallized intelligence
- memory and
- fluid intelligence (cognitive speed)

Crystallised intelligence is considered to be the cumulative total of ones acquired knowledge (i.e. wisdom of the ages such as vocabulary, overall information acquired and other knowledge-based activities). It is thought that these abilities increase up until the 6th and 7th decade of life.

Fluid intelligence, on the other hand, includes functions that are ever-changing such as planning, working memory, inhibition, mental flexibility and the initiation and monitoring of actions (Chan et al., 2008). As such, fluid intelligence is commonly referred to as **cognitive speed** (Christensen, 2003; Christensen, 2001; Reynolds, Gatz, & Pedersen, 2002). With a decline in fluid abilities comes a slower speed of information processing and slower reaction times. Therefore, decreases in these abilities are usually apparent during timed activities. These changes account for a majority of age-related cognitive changes. They may begin as early as 30 years of age, accelerating in old age (Deary et al., 2009; Greenwood & Parasurman, 2010; Park & Reuter-Lorenz, 2009; Salthouse, 2012b). For instance, cognitive speed is predicted to drop by 20% at the age of 40 years and then by 40-60% by the age of 80 years (Christensen, 2003). Research indicates that a decline in fluid abilities are experienced even in healthy older individuals, with executive functional abilities being most affected (Gunstad et al., 2006). The rate of decline, however, is dependent on many factors such as education, health, nutrition and other comorbidities (Christensen, 2001).

Memory is commonly differentiated into short-term and long-term memory, although it can also be classified into four types of memory:

- episodic memory
- semantic memory
- procedural memory and
- working memory

An example of an **episodic memory** would be a memory of your first day of school or your first kiss, episodes in your life. This type of memory is considered to decline from middle age onwards. **Semantic memory**, on the other hand, is the memory of meaning general knowledge. For example, knowing that London is the capital of the United Kingdom. This form of memory tends to increase from middle age to early young elderly and then declines after the age of 65. (Cabeza et al., 2004). **Procedural memory** is our ability to perform activities without conscious effort (e.g. how to ride a bike). These types of memories are typically preserved during healthy ageing (Ward, 2013). **Working memory** can be thought of as a temporary storage system. It can hold a limited amount of information and is used for decision making. It has been observed that this type of memory declines in older adulthood. However, some evidence suggests that the amount of decline experienced may be modulated by your sex and education (Pliatsikas, 2018)

As alluded to in the previous chapter, cognitive ageing in the brain is not only about changes in cognitive ability but adaptation to these changes (Greenwood, 2007; Loewenstein et al., 2004). Contrary to original wisdom, which once considered that lost neurons could not be replaced, it has recently been suggested that the brain network is in a permanent state of plasticity, meaning that there is the ability for nerve cells to change through new experiences even into old age. These new experiences may be related to environmental changes, learning experiences and activities, which may result in improvement in the brain's ability to structurally and functionally change and the production of new neurons (Mukadam et al., 2019; Loewestein et al., 2004; Greenwood, 2007, 2010). As such, cognitive reserve plays a vital role in off-setting neuronal loss and, by extension, cognitive decline.

Assessing changes in cognitive function can be difficult, not only from a structural point of view, because the changes can be so small, but also from a functional point of view. This is related in part to the many cognitive measures available as well as differences in administration (e.g. pencil and paper assessment versus electronic forms).

Paper tests can lead to bias and may not detect subtle changes that may be occurring. However, the development of more accurate computer-based assessments has changed this perspective in relation to evaluation. It allows for more accurate measurement of key cognitive abilities such as speed and accuracy, which are important indicators of changes in cognitive function (Pipingas et al., 2010; Salthouse, 2012a).

Changes in neurotransmitters

In Chapter 1, we discussed the value of neurotransmitters within the brain and their capacity to maintain a healthy brain. With regard to cognitive function, the key neurotransmitters to consider are serotonin and dopamine.

Serotonin is produced by nerve cells and is responsible for mood and activity. The serotonin levels can change due to age-related health and brain changes, a poor diet, chronic stress and a lack of exposure to natural light. This is important because low levels of serotonin have been associated with human depression.

On the other hand, **dopamine** is responsible for allowing you to feel pleasure, satisfaction and motivation, together with its roles in executive function, motor control, motivation and arousal, and reinforcement. This is important as dopamine levels decrease by 10% per decade of life and are associated with a decrease in cognitive functioning and motor skills. Studies in humans have demonstrated sex differences with regard to dopamine levels. For instance, dopamine levels are generally higher in females compared to males suggesting increased dopamine turnover in women due to oestrogen (Di Paolo 1994). This can therefore have important implications following menopause when levels of oestrogen decrease.

Summary

A decline in cognitive abilities is to be expected with ageing, with changes most prominent in cognitive speed/ reaction times. However, an accelerated rate of decline may indicate an increased level of neuronal damage, which may indicate neurocognitive disease. Therefore, it is important to monitor which abilities are declining and whether particular abilities are declining more rapidly than others, as this may offer clues as to whether it is associated with age-related changes or something more sinister.

CHAPTER 3:
What is Dementia?

Cognitive decline can be thought of as a sliding scale with 'normal/ optimal' cognitive function at one end and severe cognitive decline at the other. As we age, it is expected that we experience some 'normal' age-related cognitive decline due to the influence of various factors from lifestyle, genetics, ethnicity and the environment throughout our lives. In this instance, individuals will move through the scale at a slow pace, sometimes not veering too far away from their 'normal' level of cognitive functioning. However, some individuals will move through the scale more quickly due to the factors mentioned earlier, reaching **mild cognitive impairment (MCI)** or more severe forms of cognitive impairment, including dementia.

Generally, MCI is considered a precursor for dementia, and once MCI is reached, decline can be quite rapid. For instance, in 2016, it was estimated that 244 Australians progressed from MCI to dementia every day, with this number predicted to almost triple by the year 2056 (Brown et al., 2017).

Dementia is defined by the World Health Organisation (www.who.int/news-room/fact-sheets/detail/dementia) as a gradual decline in cognitive, social and physical functioning due to brain disease or damage which cannot be attributed to normal ageing (Heggie et al., 2012). Common symptoms include memory loss, impairment of perception, language, personality changes and severe cognitive decline. It is an umbrella term which can be associated with over 100 different diseases (Australian Institute of Health and Welfare, 2012 [AIHW], 2012).

It is important to understand that there are many types of dementia. Each type has different risk factors and progression of symptoms. It is also important to acknowledge that different types of dementia can co-exist, and this makes the diagnosis of dementia sub-types difficult.

The most common types of dementia are:

- Alzheimer's Disease
- Vascular dementia
- Frontotemporal dementia and
- Dementia with Lewy bodies
- (AIHW, 2012).

Unfortunately, for all types of dementia, there is currently no cure, and so symptoms are merely managed - there is no known pharmacological intervention that will inhibit the dementia process once it is initiated in the brain.

In this chapter, we will briefly discuss the distinguishing features between the different types of dementia and how dementia is diagnosed.

Alzheimer's Disease

Alzheimer's disease is a term often used interchangeably with dementia, although this is not quite correct. Alzheimer's disease is a sub-type of dementia and accounts for approximately 50-75% of Australian cases (AIHW, 2012; Blennow et al., 2006) and an estimated 50 million cases worldwide Alzheimer's disease is usually associated with ageing, with the risk increasing after 65 years of age. However, it can be sporadic and occur earlier than this.

Alzheimer's disease changes the brain in various ways. Overall, the brain is observed to shrink, which is due to the death of neurons. This is what causes the early symptoms of short-term memory loss. As the death of neurons spreads, other functions are also affected, including long-term memory, emotional regulation, social skills and speed (Buckner, 2004).

A hallmark of Alzheimer's disease is the deposit of a protein referred to as **amyloid**. These deposits build up over time in organs such as the brain, which can cause damage and impair signalling of the neurons. In addition, Alzheimer's disease is also associated with **neurofibrillary tangles**. These kill the neurons by starving them of resources (Prince et al., 2014).

Vascular dementia

As the name suggests, **vascular dementia** is caused by problems with the vascular system and blood supply to the brain. A number of lifestyle factors that are associated with increased stress on the heart and a reduction of blood flow increase the risk for vascular dementia.

There are two sub-types of vascular dementia; **multi-infarct dementia** and **Binswanger's disease** (also known as **subcortical vascular dementia**). Multi-infarct dementia is the more common of the two and is caused by infarcts or strokes (Prince et al., 2014). An **infarct** is a disruption of blood flow to the brain, which can be due to a clot, haemorrhage or narrowing of the arteries. Over time, the damage caused by multiple infarcts spreads, causing damage to areas of the brain. As such, symptoms may progress more slowly than Alzheimer's disease but may also include epilepsy (Prince et al., 2014).

Binswanger's disease is similar to multi-infarct dementia. It is also caused by disruptions to blood flow to various parts of the brain. However, changes associated with Binswanger's disease often occur deep within the brain in the white matter. Early symptoms can include lethargy, impaired cognition, difficulty walking, emotional dysregulation and lack of bladder control, as the white matter is responsible for effective transmission of signalling for these functions (Libon et al., 1990).

Lewy Body dementia

Lewy body dementia is the second most common form of degenerative dementia behind Alzheimer's disease. Similar to Alzheimer's disease, Lewy body dementia is associated with the death of brain cells. The death of these brain cells is thought to be related to changes inside the nerve cells due to an abnormal volume of protein molecules called alpha-synuclein, referred to as Lewy bodies (AIHW, 2012). It is also thought that Lewy bodies may contribute to Parkinson's disease.

The progression of Lewy body dementia is quite rapid. Symptoms include difficulties in concentration, memory loss, confusion and difficulties judging distance. However, what distinguishes it from other types of dementia, is the presence of at least two of the following:

- Visual hallucinations
- Tremors or muscle stiffness/ rigidity
- Fluctuation in orientation and mental state

The symptoms of Lewy body dementia can be difficult to treat due to an overlap between symptoms of other conditions such as Parkinson's disease and the effects of medications on other symptoms of the disease. For instance, some medications used in Parkinson's patients to reduce tremors can make the hallucinations experienced in Lewy body dementia worse, while some anti-hallucination medications can increase the severity of tremors and muscle rigidity (Boot et al., 2013).

Frontotemporal dementia

As discussed in chapter 1, the frontal lobes are associated with executive functions, including planning, judgement, mood, and self-control. On the other hand, the temporal lobes are associated with processing visual and auditory information-making sense of what we see and what we hear. As the name suggests, **frontotemporal dementia** is associated with progressive damage to these areas of the brain. This is thought to be related to a build-up of two types of protein that accumulate in brain cells in FTD–tau and TDP-43, leading to the death of the cells and shrinkage of the brain over time. As such, symptoms include changes in personality and behaviour and declines in language skills (AIHW, 2012; Economics, 2009; Prince et al., 2014).

Whether the frontal or temporal lobes are affected first will determine what sub-type of frontotemporal dementia is diagnosed. If frontal lobes are affected first, this is referred to as **behaviour-variant frontotemporal dementia**, reflecting changes observed in behaviour and personality. Specifically, this can include changes in emotional response and behaviour, loss of inhibition, impulsiveness, changes in eating patterns and a decline in self-care (Dementia Australia, 2000).

If the temporal lobes are affected first, this will either be classified as **semantic dementia** or **progressive non-fluent aphasia** (Dementia Australia, 2000). Referring back to chapter 2, semantic memory refers to knowledge of the meaning of words, objects and concepts. Therefore, in semantic dementia, this knowledge becomes impaired, leading to difficulties in assigning meaning to words, forgetting people's names and finding the right words to explain what they mean. In contrast, in progressive non-fluent aphasia, communication becomes difficult as the production of speech is affected. These individuals may slur their words, have distorted speech, and may experience difficulties in reading and spelling. However, this is the least common form of frontotemporal dementia and is often seen in older individuals (Dementia Australia, 2000).

Unlike Alzheimer's disease, memory is often not affected in the early stages of frontotemporal dementia. However, frontotemporal dementia often affects people at younger ages than Alzheimer's disease, with symptoms typically beginning from the age of 50 (Dementia Australia, 2000).

Younger-onset dementia

Although the risk for dementia generally increases with age, younger individuals can also be diagnosed. **Younger-onset dementia** is the term used for anyone diagnosed with dementia before the age of 65. Younger-onset dementia includes the types of dementia described above, although symptoms can occur in individuals as young as 30. According to Dementia Australia, in 2019, 27,247 Australians were living with younger-onset dementia.

Younger-onset dementia is relatively rare. However, it can be difficult to diagnose as it can be caused by other rare and unfamiliar medical conditions. The symptoms can be different when compared to symptoms displayed by older individuals with dementia (Dementia Australia, 2016).

How is dementia diagnosed?

Given there is often an overlap of symptoms and subtypes of dementia, no single test can be used to diagnose dementia. Therefore, a comprehensive review of past and family medical history in conjunction with a range of clinical assessments are often used, including:

- Medical Imaging (CT, MRI, PET)- to detect changes in the structure of the brain
- Blood tests
- Cognitive assessments- to detect changes in memory and other cognitive skills
- Lumbar puncture (cerebral spinal fluid testing)
- Autopsy

Due to the nature of the changes which occur in some types of dementia, a diagnosis can sometimes only be reached after death during an autopsy. For example, changes observed in Lewy body dementia can only be seen by examining the brain cells, which can only be done after death.

Diagnosis of dementia also often occurs when the disease has already progressed due to the common misconception that symptoms are just a part of normal ageing. Although there is no cure available, there are treatments to manage the symptoms to improve the quality of life, so early diagnosis is beneficial. Early diagnosis can also increase the ability to plan for disease progression. The person can actively participate in the decision-making process regarding their care when the disease progresses to advanced stages. Therefore, it is important to recognise potential early symptoms of dementia and to visit your doctor if you are concerned. You can find a checklist of early symptoms, more information and support services on the Dementia Australia website (www.dementia.org.au).

CHAPTER 4:

How does lifestyle impact brain ageing?

While people generally have an idea about what behaviours are healthy for them, many lifestyle factors which contribute to maintaining cognitive function into old age are often overlooked ((NHMRC), 2014; Arab & Sabbagh, 2010; Barnes & Yaffe, 2011; Gatz et al., 2006; Hultsch, 1999; Laurin et al., 2001; Lautenschlager et al., 2012). This chapter will provide a brief overview of some of the main factors that research has identified as important and how they contribute to better brain health.

Exercise

It is generally accepted that exercise is good for the brain. But there are many different types of exercise, and so the question becomes, what type of exercise is best? In this section, we will discuss some of the main types of exercise and how they are thought to affect the brain. However, it is important to note that you should **not** begin any new exercise regime without first consulting your medical practitioner.

Aerobic

Aerobic exercise includes activities that increase your heart rate and your breathing. This can include swimming, power-walking, running or cycling. There is considerable evidence indicating that regular aerobic training is associated with improved cognitive function. It may slow or even prevent age-related cognitive decline, even in high-risk individuals (e.g. those who have a genetic risk for dementia) (Ahlskog et al., 2011; Colcombe & Kramer, 2003; Cotman & Berchtold, 2002; Cotman et al., 2007; Dalgas et al., 2013; Davenport et al., 2012; Deslandes et al., 2009; Gates et al., 2011; Hultsch et al., 1999; Knöchel et al., 2012; Larson & Bruce, 1987; Matta Mello Portugal et al., 2013; Netz et al., 2005; Ni et al., 2011; Okoro et al., 2013; Voss et al., 2011; Wang et al., 2013). Improvements in overall cognitive function, memory and executive functioning have all been reported following aerobic training. In some cases, aerobic training has been found to reverse cognitive decline in those with dementia (Heyn et al., 2004).

While there are vast differences in the research regarding how much aerobic exercise we should do to reap these benefits, it appears that it comes down to how the exercise impacts our **aerobic fitness**. This is our heart's ability to send oxygen to our muscles. Given that the brain uses 25% of the body's overall oxygen consumption, it is not surprising that an improvement in the body's ability to get oxygen to the brain may be behind the cognitive benefits of aerobic exercise.

So, how can you tell if your aerobic fitness is improving? Research suggests that improvements in aerobic fitness may be reflected by a slower resting heart rate and a reduction in heart rate over time when performing a particular exercise at a particular intensity. For instance, if you begin a regime of running 2km every day at a moderate intensity at the beginning of March, your heart rate at the end of the same run six weeks later may be lower - this may reflect an improvement in aerobic fitness.

Resistance Training

Resistance or **strength training** refers to exercise which improves your muscular strength and endurance. Activities including lifting weights or using resistance bands are considered to be resistance training exercises.

Research investigating whether resistance training can be beneficial for your brain is relatively new; however, there are promising findings. For instance, studies have reported improvements in various fields, including global cognitive function, memory, executive function and attention (Anderson-Hanley et al., 2010; Best et al., 2015; Cassilhas et al., 2007; de Camargo, 2016; Ikudome et al., 2016; Liu-Ambrose et al., 2010; Liu-Ambrose et al., 2012), with some improvements even reported in those who are cognitively impaired (Bolandzadeh et al., 2015; Suo et al., 2016).

Improvements in cognitive function due to resistance training are thought to occur due to a link between muscles and the brain. When muscle strength or muscle mass increases, there are associated increases in various blood markers. These blood markers can cross the blood-brain barrier and may have positive effects on cognition.

The American College of Sports Medicine (https://www. acsm.org/) has published guidelines regarding how much resistance training is needed for older adults in order to build muscle mass and strength, given muscle mass tends to naturally decline with age. However, given research into the effects of resistance training on cognition is so new, and there are many different individual factors which can contribute to determining how much exercise one should do, it is unclear how much resistance training can produce cognitive benefits. However, the majority of the current research which have reported positive effects have used moderate-intensity exercise programs, which were conducted a couple of times a week.

Tai-chi

Tai-chi is characterised by choreographed patterns of movement which incorporate cognitive, social and meditation skills. It is considered an alternative type of aerobic exercise and is normally regarded as a moderate-intensity activity. Research has found that tai-chi is effective for maintaining global cognitive function and may even be more effective than simply doing physical activities (Lim et al., 2019). It has also been found to be effective for improving cognitive function in older adults in the early stages of dementia (Lim et al., 2019).

It is believed that due to the aerobic nature of tai-chi, the increased blood circulation may promote cognitive benefits through increased oxygen supply to the brain. Furthermore, in combination with meditation, the relaxation and stress reduction which comes from practising tai-chi may also account for its cognitive benefits (Siu & Lee, 2018). Lastly, given that tai-chi requires learning a series of choreographed movements requiring attention and executive function, the cognitive stimulation achieved through tai-chi may also explain its perceived benefits (Siu & Lee, 2018).

Multi-component exercise

It is evident from the information above that different types of exercise appear to benefit the brain through different pathways. This then begs the question, is it better to participate in a program that incorporates multiple types of exercise rather than a single modality exercise program to maximise cognitive benefits?

Overall, the findings are mixed, although there is some evidence suggesting that multi-component exercise is more beneficial for cognitive function than single modality exercise (Colcombe & Kramer, 2003), even in those who are cognitively impaired (Heyn et al., 2004). Despite this, the take-home message regarding exercise is that most studies have found that some exercise, regardless of type, results in improvements in cognitive function compared to those who don't exercise at all.

Diet

This section will be covered in more detail later, but briefly, research supports that there are particular foods containing nutrients which are good for the brain. These nutrients include antioxidants, B vitamins, vitamin D and other vitamins (e.g. vitamin A, C and E), saturated and trans fats, omega-3 fatty acids and polyphenols. Foods rich in these nutrients generally fit into a **Mediterranean style diet** which is characterised by a high intake of fruits, vegetables, legumes, nuts and fish; a high intake of unsaturated fatty acids (Kiefte-de Jong et al., 2014; Ortega et al., 1997; Samieri et al., 2013). In particular, green leafy vegetables have been found to be particularly beneficial for cognitive function as they are rich in vitamins such as vitamin C and K and carotenoids, which act as an antioxidant.

In contrast, foods high in animal and saturated fats and refined sugars have been associated with poorer cognitive function (Cordain et al., 2005; Kanoski & Davidson, 2011; Solfrizzi et al.). A dietary pattern which is high in the intake of these foods combined with a low intake of the healthy foods listed above is typically known as a **Western-style diet.** The high intake of fats and sugars associated with this diet can contribute to high cholesterol and heart problems which, in turn, can lead to increases in pro-inflammatory markers in the blood. This increase in inflammation can cause oxidative stress, which, as mentioned earlier, can have detrimental impacts on the brain. Due to an increase in cholesterol, the arteries may also begin to narrow due to the build-up of plaque which can reduce the efficiency of blood flow and, thus, oxygen to the brain.

As stated above, there is evidence to suggest that increases in muscle mass or strength may also be associated with improvements in cognitive function due to resistance training. In order to promote muscle growth, it is important that we consume adequate amounts of protein, particularly if participating in resistance training. This is especially important for older adults as our protein requirements increase as we age.

Protein can come from many different sources (e.g. soy protein, supplements, animal protein, plant protein etc.), and the research is unclear whether any particular source is more beneficial than another. However, if consuming animal protein (meat), it is important that the meat is lean, unprocessed meat (such as lean cuts of veal), as processed meats (such as salami etc.), can have a higher salt content which can contribute to negative effects on cardiovascular health.

Alcohol

There is currently insufficient and inconsistent research on the effects of alcohol on brain health. However, there is consistent evidence that excessive alcohol consumption can lead to cognitive decline. For instance, a condition referred to as **Korsakoff's syndrome**, which is characterised as a memory disorder due to a severe thiamine (vitamin B-1) deficiency, is often related to alcohol misuse, although there can be other causes.

It is thought that alcohol may negatively impact the brain due to the toxic effects that alcohol has on a cell level. Even in moderate drinkers (those who drink occasionally), when ingested, alcohol is converted by the body into a highly toxic substance referred to as acetaldehyde which can have direct effects on organs, including the brain (Manzo-Avalos & Saavedra-Molina, 2010). Further, repeated intoxication and hangovers can also increase the stress experienced in the body, which can negatively impact the brain. Lastly, inebriation can lead to an increased risk for falls or injury, which may result in a head injury. Depending on the severity of the fall and injury, this can have lifelong impacts on brain function.

Stress

Stress can be thought of as a bell-shaped curve- that is, when your stress levels are too low or too high, your performance is likely to be negatively affected. But when you have an 'optimal' amount of stress, your performance is likely to be at its best. This is known as the **Yerkes-Dodson Law**. This section will focus on when stress levels are too high and how this can impact the brain, as this is when cognitive function is usually negatively impacted.

When faced with a stressful situation, particular parts of your brain have less energy and resources available to them as your brain goes into a 'survival mode', activating essential parts of the brain to deal with the stressor. This can have a detrimental impact on various aspects of cognition, including memory and attention, as these parts of the brain are considered less crucial than others when fighting a stressor (Yaribeygi et al., 2017).

If you experience stress over a long period of time (chronic stress), this can ultimately lead to a 'rewiring' of your brain. This occurs through a loss of neurons and neurodegeneration (Yaribeygi et al., 2017). For instance, it has been found that in those who experience chronic stress, the parts of the brain which are initiated during 'survival mode' are more active than those which are not (memory and attention), leading to a long-term impact on these cognitive functions (Bottaccioli et al., 2019; Yaribeygi et al., 2017). You can think of the parts of your brain like a muscle in this scenario. The parts that are being used actively (the survival parts) are being exercised more and so more neural connections are made, strengthening the networks in these areas. In contrast, areas of the brain which are not being allocated resources and which are not being used as much, such as those responsible for memory and executive function, begin to get weaker as their neural connections are lost due to neurodegeneration.

Not all stress is considered the same, and there are several factors that have been suggested to determine whether there will be detrimental impacts on the brain. These include:

- If the stress was unpredicted - e.g. the sudden death of a spouse. This type of stress may be more damaging as you haven't had time to prepare for or to begin processing the stress.

- There is no perceived time limit on the stress - stressors which are often related to a particular event are usually perceived as less damaging as an individual knows that the stress will come to an end (e.g. an exam).
- Lack of support - those who do not feel supported during times of stress will often experience greater cognitive impacts.

The best thing you can do with regard to stress is to manage it appropriately. There are many different ways that you can do this, although research generally supports positive effects of the following:

- Getting enough sleep - sleep can assist in the regeneration of the areas of the brain which may be depleted of resources
- Mindfulness or relaxation techniques to reduce the stress
- Maintaining a healthy diet which may reduce oxidative reactions caused by stress
- Exercise - this can help use up some of that unhelpful nervous energy, can increase endorphins (the good stuff!) and may be used as a distraction
- Seek support/ help if needed
- Remain positive - try to perceive the stress as a learning experience

Smoking

Cigarettes are often used as a form of stress relief. While smoking may be perceived to reduce stress levels in some individuals, it can also harm your brain and put you at a higher risk for dementia (Deal et al., 2020; R. Peters et al., 2008).

Quitting smoking is one of the best things you can do to improve your brain health. This is due to the positive effects on other organs, including your heart and lungs, which, as we already know, play a big role in providing oxygen to the brain. For instance, when you smoke, you are inhaling carbon monoxide, which counteracts the oxygen in your body. According to the smokefree.gov website (https://smokefree. gov/ 2021), smoking also increases the stress on your heart by changing the consistency of your blood, making it more difficult for your heart to pump around the body. It can also increase fatty deposits inside your arteries which can lead to blood clots, affecting blood flow. Therefore, by decreasing and quitting your smoking, you can avoid these outcomes, which can negatively affect the brain.

However, it is important to acknowledge that quitting smoking is not easy and that you may need assistance or multiple attempts to succeed. This is because smoking changes your brain. In order to accommodate for the large doses of nicotine you inhale when you smoke, your brain creates additional nicotine receptors. These additional receptors are what cause the cravings and withdrawal symptoms when you try to quit. Therefore, nicotine replacement therapy is often used as a safe alternative for cigarettes when trying to quit smoking. The nicotine from this therapy locks onto the nicotine receptors, allowing the craving to pass.

Sleep

Sleep is a vital function necessary for survival. In fact, we spend roughly one-third of our lives sleeping. Our bodies use this time to grow and repair tissues, to synthesise hormones and to restore energy. With regard to the brain, neurons are re-organised, and waste products that have been created during the day are eliminated. As a result, information is moved from short-term memory into long-term memory. Activity in areas of the brain associated with emotional regulation is also increased, allowing these areas to maintain adaptive behaviours while you are awake and when faced with stressors.

There are four different stages of sleep. The amount of time spent in each stage can determine how well your body and brain repairs itself during this time which can influence how you feel when you wake up in the morning.

- *Stage 1: non-rapid eye movement (REM) sleep:* In the first 7 minutes of falling asleep, you are in a light sleep. During this stage, your brain waves, eye movements, and heart rate slow down.

- *Stage 2:* Following the first 7 minutes, your body temperature decreases, your eye movements stop, and your heart rate and muscles relax. Your brain waves spike and then slow down again. This is the stage where you spend most of your sleep.

- *Rapid eye movement (REM) sleep:* this occurs roughly 90 minutes after falling asleep. This is typically when dreaming occurs as this is when your brain is organising information, which is essential for learning and memory

- ***Stage 3 and 4:*** is deep sleep. This is when restoration happens - your eyes and muscles don't move, and your brain waves are at their slowest.

As we age, the amount of sleep we need changes. Younger children and teenagers require the most amount of sleep as this is the time when the most growth occurs in the body. For an adult, between 7 and 9 hours a night is recommended. For older adults, this reduces to 7 to 8 hours as functions begin to slow down and which therefore require less energy and restoration.

It is important to note that if you are consistently not meeting your sleep requirements, this can lead to a **sleep debt**, thereby increasing risks for a number of health problems as your body has less time to repair itself. Unfortunately, the fix for chronic sleep debt is not as simple as sleeping in longer on the weekend (although this is fine if you have had a pretty average sleep the night before). In fact, one study found that it can take four days to recover from one hour of missed sleep (Kitamura et al., 2016). Therefore, a consistent sleep routine where you go to bed and get up at the same time every day is beneficial for maintaining good sleep quantity and quality.

Despite this, it is not uncommon for older adults to have complaints regarding their sleep quality and getting to sleep, especially in those with mild cognitive impairment (Falck et al., 2018). This is important as sleep quality has been linked to dementia and cognitive decline (Falck et al., 2018).

There are a number of approaches that can be taken to improve sleep quality, although these should be discussed with your doctor as the most effective approach may depend on the cause of the sleep disturbance. For instance, sleep can be disturbed for multiple reasons, including getting up to go to the bathroom, stress, sleep hygiene, insomnia, medication side effects etc. Thus, the appropriate treatment for sleep disturbance related to stress may be different to that recommended for the side effects of medication.

However, briefly, some of the approaches often used to improve sleep quality with good effect can include:

- Modification to physical activity
- Relaxation and stress-reduction techniques
- Bright light therapy
- Melatonin supplementation
- Changes to sleep hygiene
- Changes to medications

'Brain training'- cognitive stimulation

Thanks to brain plasticity, the more we engage our brain in new and cognitively stimulating activities, the more neural connections are formed and strengthened, thereby increasing our cognitive reserve. There is an abundance of research to support that engaging in activities such as **brain training** or **cognitive training** (particularly when combined with other interventions such as exercise) can help to maintain and improve cognitive function across the lifespan, even in those with mild cognitive impairment (ÇInar & Sahiner, 2020; Miotto et al., 2018; Pappas & Drigas, 2019; Sittiprapaporn, 2020; Takeuchi et al., 2020).

It is thought that restoring areas of the brain by re-engaging them by doing activities that are cognitively challenging or even new (e.g. beginning a new hobby) can restore lost neurons in areas of the brain that were used more actively in the past or can create new connections in areas of the brain that were not used as much. When combined with activities such as exercise, which can help to promote these new connections, the effects of brain training may be magnified.

Summary

Overall, it is evident that by maintaining a healthy lifestyle and keeping your mind active, you can naturally assist your body in maintaining brain health and cognitive function throughout the lifespan. Given that there are several mechanisms through which each lifestyle factor influences your brain, a combination of all of the above may be the best to achieve maximal retention of cognitive function into old age.

CHAPTER 5:
Myths and Truths

In this chapter, we address many common myths associated with cognitive ageing and dementia. We consider the research and aim to provide a summary of the current knowledge.

Myth: Everyone will eventually get dementia due to old age.

Truth: Though the risk for dementia increases with age, this does not mean that everyone will get dementia. Indeed, the most common form of Alzheimer's disease is late-onset dementia which refers to the development of symptoms after the age of 65. However, it is estimated that 5% of the population may develop early-onset dementia (Ferri et al., 2005).

Differences in the formation of plaque and changes which occur in the brain are somewhat dependent on when the symptoms occur, and this suggests that ageing is not the only risk factor for dementia. Therefore, there are many other factors to consider rather than just ageing. For instance, the Ferri study considered the influence of genetic predisposition. Data from 3403 individuals from 1492 families showed that age at symptom onset and death of people with genetic frontotemporal dementia was influenced by their genetic group, particularly genetic mutations found in their family. This suggests that DNA from other family members may be particularly helpful in individuals with genetic mutations specifically. Consider changing to Microtubule Associated Protein Tau (MAPT). The MAPT gene provides instructions for making a protein called tau, which is commonly found to build up in the brain in certain types of dementia.

So, overall, though your risk generally increases the older that you get,. The risk may be increased depending on your genetics.

Myth: People who have had a stroke will get dementia.

Truth: A stroke occurs when there is a sudden change in the blood supply to the brain. Many strokes are caused by the blocking of arteries leading to the brain (ischemic stroke). Other strokes are caused by bleeding into brain tissue when a blood vessel bursts (haemorrhagic stroke). As a stroke occurs rapidly and requires immediate treatment, stroke may be referred to as a 'brain attack'. When the symptoms of a stroke last only a short time (less than an hour), this is called a transient ischemic attack (TIA) or a mini-stroke.

Given reduced blood supply for even a short period of time can impact the survival and recovery of brain tissue, it is not surprising that the current research does indeed suggest that the risk for dementia is higher following a stroke (Gorelick, 2018; Yeh et al., 2019). However, this does not necessarily mean that all stroke victims will go on to develop dementia. There are a number of other factors which can contribute to this risk, as well as a number of actions which can be taken to reduce this risk.

Research indicates that the likelihood of cognitive impairment due to stroke may be associated with a recurrence of ischemic stroke in high-risk patients. In such cases, anti-blocking agents are required to clear the arteries to reduce the reoccurrence of stroke and, thus, cognitive impairment and risk for dementia (Bunch et al., 2020; Goulay et al., 2020; Kwon et al., 2020).

Stroke rehabilitation programs also offer a way to regain/improve skills which may have been affected by the stroke. These aim to recover, repair or replace, and rebuild/re-strengthen neuronal pathways in the brain which may have been damaged. Given this damage may be repaired, this is protective against the development of dementia later on. This is supported by one study conducted by Yi-Chun and colleagues (2012), which found that rehabilitation following ischemic stroke reduced the risk for dementia compared to those who did not receive rehabilitation. Similarly, another study found that the earlier stroke rehabilitation was undertaken, the better the outcomes (Mukamal et al., 2003). It is important to note, however, that in this study, they found that recovery was largely dependent on the severity and type of cognitive impairment suffered, as well as the age of the stroke victim (Mukamal et al., 2003).

Myth: Having bad teeth increases the risk for dementia.

Truth: It is important to begin by saying that it is not really the health of your teeth that impacts your risk for your dementia. Instead, the health of your teeth is likely to reflect the healthiness of your overall lifestyle, which may contribute to your risk of developing dementia. As such, the published research does not focus on bad dentition; rather, it has considered tooth loss and periodontal disease (infections of the structures around the teeth, which include the gums, periodontal ligament and alveolar bone).

With respect to tooth loss, a review conducted in 2018 suggested that loss of teeth may be associated with an increased risk for dementia. However, further well-designed studies need to be completed (Fang et al., 2018). Regarding periodontal disease, several recent studies suggest that there is a causal relationship between periodontal disease and dementia. It is thought that this may also be associated with the socio-economic condition in which the individual is living. Those living in low socioeconomic areas may be more likely to suffer periodontal disease due to other related conditions and lifestyle habits, including smoking, diabetes, poor diet and overall poor oral hygiene (Choi et al., 2019; Orr et al., 2020; Pazos et al., 2018; Yoo et al., 2019).

Myth: Intellectual disabilities increase the risk for dementia.

Truth: Assessing cognitive function in individuals with intellectual disability can prove difficult due to the nature of testing and the populations to which standardised tests are pitched. While an intellectual disability indicates that there are areas of the brain which are not fully developed, current research does not indicate that a person with an intellectual disability has any greater chance of developing dementia than a non-intellectually impaired person (Kuske & Muller, 2017; Lucock et al., 2019; McKenzie et al., 2018; Ward & Parkes, 2017).

Myth: Head injuries lead to dementia.

Truth: A recent study using MRI investigated injured areas of the brain in individuals who had previously experienced a traumatic brain injury. This study concluded that areas of brain atrophy (a loss of neurons and the connections between them) may be subject to cognitive impairment. However, if the hippocampus (memory centre of the brain) is unaffected, then the potential for dementia is reduced (Meysami et al., 2019). In contrast, if one experiences craniofacial trauma (injury of the face or skull), there is an increased risk of dementia. This may be related to the areas of the brain that are likely to be affected and the functions they are responsible for (Schneider et al., 2019; Yang et al., 2019). Therefore, it is important to acknowledge that the severity and location of the injury may play a role in determining the risk for the development of cognitive impairment leading to dementia (Arulsamy et al., 2019; Elder et al., 2019; Hicks et al., 2019).

Myth: Chronic depression, anxiety, or stress increases the risk for dementia.

Truth: There are a number of environmental factors which may influence mood as we age (Voros et al., 2020). Depression, anxiety, and chronic stress can all substantially impact well-being and, in some instances, cognitive function. However, the association between each of these factors and the risk for dementia needs to be considered independently.

Research does suggest that there is an association between depression and an increased risk for dementia (Bennet, 2013; Cherbuin et al., 2015). However, some research suggests that this is mainly associated with depression earlier in life rather than late life (Byers et al., 2011). In contrast, other research suggests that the risk for dementia due to depression in late life is just as significant, possibly predicting a two-fold increase in the risk for dementia (Cherbuin et al., 2015). Therefore, while it is considered that depression may increase the risk for dementia, the risk may be dependent on the age of onset of depression.

With regard to anxiety, one study which looked at twins found that those who experienced chronic high anxiety at any time had a 48% greater risk for dementia than their identical twin (Petkus et al., 2015). However, other research suggests that there is no association between anxiety and anxiety disorders and the risk for dementia (de Bruijn et al., 2015). Therefore, the risk may be related to coping strategies and resilience, which may ultimately impact the physical toll that this stress has on your body, although this is not currently clear.

There are many factors that can produce stress as we age. These can include changes in one's environment (i.e. your home or living facility), the onset of new health conditions or deterioration in existing health conditions, death of a spouse or friends, as well as changes in employment (i.e. retirement) which may impact finances. Stress, particularly chronic stress, can significantly impact various organs including the brain due to inflammation in the body. Therefore, it is not surprising that research suggests that there may be some relationship between stress and dementia. Specifically, research suggests that work-related stress, particularly in mid-life, may be associated with an increased risk for dementia (Sindi et al., 2017; Wong et al., 2015).

Myth: Untreated high blood pressure increases the risk for dementia.

Truth: High blood pressure (hypertension) is generally considered any measurement of more than 140/90 millimetres of mercury. Low blood pressure (hypotension) is defined as less than 90/60 millimetres of mercury.

High blood pressure may be a genetic abnormality, although it is commonly a result of inadequate exercise and poor diet. As we age, systolic blood pressure (the top number) generally increases, while diastolic (the bottom number) can decrease due to structural changes in the blood vessels in the brain. A recent study which evaluated data from more than 4,700 participants collected over 25 years in the US reported that those with high blood pressure during middle age and during late life were 49% more likely to develop dementia than those with normal blood pressure. Furthermore, being hypertensive in middle age and then hypotensive in late-life, increased dementia risk by 62% (Walker et al., 2019). Consistent with this, another independent study of 5,273 participants concluded that if there is a large blood pressure variation over a period of years, the long-term risk for dementia was increased (Ma et al., 2019). Therefore, it is also important to be mindful of low blood pressure, which can arise due to the stiffening or hardening of the arteries related to disease and physical frailty. On the flip side, low blood pressure may be a consequence of dementia as it may disrupt the brain's nervous system.

Together, this evidence suggests that you should have your blood pressure checked regularly by your doctor. If it is abnormal, beginning medication to normalise it may reduce your risk for dementia later in life.

Myth: High cholesterol increases the risk of dementia.

Truth: Research suggests that in non-demented older adults, high serum cholesterol is associated with disruption of functional connectivity within the networks of the brain (Spielberg et al., 2017). This suggests that high cholesterol accelerates the impact of ageing on neural pathways in the brain by disrupting connectivity in circuits implicated in integrative processes and behavioural control (Spielberg et al., 2017; Zhang et al., 2016). With regard to Alzheimer's disease, the impact of serum cholesterol and how it may be associated with neuropathology has been demonstrated by evidence derived from genetic, epidemiological, and biochemical studies. There is evidence that cholesterol can significantly influence amyloid-beta (Ab) production, which results in the formation of amyloid plaques within blood vessels which are the hallmark of dementia.

Together, this suggests that careful and regular monitoring of your cholesterol levels should be conducted with your doctor. If your cholesterol is high, lifestyle changes can be put in place to manage your levels, although some people may require medication.

Myth: Obesity increases the risk for dementia.

Truth: Obesity is commonly defined as a body mass index (BMI) of 30 or more. According to research, obesity may indirectly influence cognition through vascular risk factors or through direct effects of adipocyte-derived hormones. The main role of these hormones in the body is to function as a fuel tank for the storage of other mechanisms which can influence cognitive function (Cho et al., 2018).

When considering obesity, it is important to evaluate where your weight is carried as this can affect your risk for dementia. For instance, a recent study highlighted that late-life central obesity (weight carried around your middle) was positively associated with the development of dementia in older persons (Choi et al., 2019). Similarly, a large meta-analysis consisting of 2.8 million adults with 57,294 cases of dementia from 19 cohort studies evaluated the relationship of BMI, waist circumference, and annual percent weight change with risk of dementia (Lee & Choi, 2019). Obesity was associated with a higher risk for vascular dementia, while weight gain was only slightly associated with higher vascular dementia risk. Lastly, a 10-year population-based study of 478 individuals aged 65 and over found that in individuals younger than 88 years with central obesity, even modest degrees of high cholesterol might independently predispose them to faster cognitive decline than those younger than 87 years without central obesity (Ganguli et al., 2020). Therefore, other physiological factors that may occur concurrently with obesity are also important to consider as they can further increase your risk.

Taken together, this suggests that the higher your BMI, the higher the risk for dementia. However, it is essential to point out that BMI can be impacted by muscle weight. For instance, bodybuilders often have a high BMI. However, this does not increase their risk for dementia as they are generally very conscious of their health habits and their BMI is not reflective of excess adiposity. Thus, it is important to consider where your weight is carried and what type of weight it is (i.e. muscle versus fat). Further, it is important to acknowledge that the relationship between body size, weight change, and dementia is complex and exhibits non-linear associations depending on the dementia subtype (Lee et al., 2019).

Myth: Heart attacks increase the risk for dementia.

Truth: Heart disease is a frequent cause of cerebral compromise. However, data concerning heart-brain disorders relating to the associated complications of dementia are rare (Finsterer & Stollberger, 2016).

Among patients with heart failure, transient neurological attacks (TNAs) can occur, indicating the presence of cerebrovascular disease. These attacks usually last for less than 24 hours. They can include changes in vision, slurred speech, weakness or paralysis in parts of the body and difficulties with balance. As these attacks are associated with brief disruptions to blood flow, they are also considered to be associated with an increased risk for cognitive impairment, which may suggest that these attacks are associated with an increased risk of future dementia.

Reductions in blood flow which often lead to a heart attack may be caused by the closure of the arteries. This is due to atherosclerosis which are deposits of fats, cholesterol and other substances in and on your artery walls (plaque), which can restrict blood flow. This plaque build-up can explode, which triggers a blood clot. Alternatively, clots that restrict the amount of blood flow and oxygen to the brain over a long period of time may increase the risk for dementia by depriving the brain of these valuable resources required for plasticity and neuronal connections. There is a need for more clinical awareness of this problem and it needs to be investigated with more research.

Myth: Kidney disease increases the risk for dementia.

Truth: Chronic kidney disease has been demonstrated to exhibit significant premature ageing characteristics in many different organ systems, including the brain (Chiu et al., 2019). As such, cognitive impairment is commonly found in patients with chronic kidney disease (Yeh et al., 2019).

In a 2-year prospective cohort study of 131 pre-dialysis chronic kidney disease patients aged 65 years and over, cognitive impairment was common (Yeh et al., 2019). Given that incidences of depression are also quite high in these patients, this may further contribute to the risk for cognitive impairment.

In patients undergoing dialysis, it has been estimated that between 16 and 38% have cognitive impairment, including dementia. This is approximately three times higher than the value observed in age-matched non-chronic kidney diseased individuals (Joseph et al., 2019). This manifests as accumulative neuron damage, which, as research suggests, is a precursor commonly occurring many years before clinical cognitive impairment or dementia (Chiu et al., 2019). However, it has been suggested that cognitive impairment in these patients is also affected by other demographic factors, which are commonly associated with cognitive decline as well as the duration of dialysis (Joseph et al., 2019).

Myth: My ethnicity increases the risk for dementia.

Truth: Race and ethnicity are among the risk factors which are considered to be important as they may include considerations around differences in lifestyle, health and socioeconomic status, which also contribute to risk. Current research estimates that the global prevalence of dementia in individuals aged 56 years and over is 5-7%, with a higher prevalence in Latin America (Mukadam et al., 2019).

Particular research has focused on memory and visuospatial decline between ethnic groups. This research suggests that it is important to examine the interactions between race/ethnicity and sex/gender to give a greater understanding of cognitive ageing disparities and lead to the development of more targeted ways to prevent or slow cognitive decline (Avila et al., 2019). Another study conducted in the United States which evaluated 771 dementia cases, found that dementia rates were lowest among an Asian population followed by Caucasian, Latinos and non-Caucasian populations (Gilsanz et al., 2019). However, this may be a by-product of a lack of awareness and cultural norms around mental health and dementia in some populations, which may artificially lower the rate of dementia in these groups (Fletcher 2020).

Myth: Where I live in the world will determine my risk for dementia.

Truth: As stated above, ethnicity may impact your risk for dementia. However, we recognise that many people may live in countries in which they were not born. So this myth becomes more about environmental differences between countries and regions in the world.

Research suggests that those who live in areas where they have exposure to lead or other heavy metals have an increased risk for age-related decline (Moon et al., 2019). Those who live in low socio-economic areas where access to education may be more limited than in other areas may also experience an increased risk for cognitive decline and dementia due to having a lower cognitive reserve (Luth et al., 2019). Those living in these areas may also struggle with access to healthcare facilities and may not be able to afford to maintain a healthy lifestyle through nutritious foods and exercise, which, as we know, can impact the risk for dementia. However, the quality of evidence surrounding this issue is quite low and further studies are needed.

Myth: My sex suggests that I am more likely to get dementia.

Truth: The available research suggests that two out of every three Alzheimer's patients are female and that postmenopausal women represent over 60% of these cases (Rahman et al., 2019). One explanation is the **oestrogen hypothesis**. During menopause, women experience a decrease in oestrogen. Given oestrogen can increase cerebral blood flow, display anti-inflammatory properties and enhance neural activity, a decrease in this hormone may contribute to cognitive decline. Therefore, men who do not experience a change in oestrogen levels have a lower risk.

As we know, it is not only biology that impacts risk, and so changes and differences in social activity, mental health, marital status, and lifestyle also need to be considered as well as sex when predicting risk for dementia (Rahman et al., 2019). Given that women typically live longer than men, they may experience more of these changes, which may induce stress, anxiety, depression, and more health conditions, thereby increasing their risk.

Myth: The more medication I take, the greater my risk for dementia.

Truth: Ageing is associated with a number of chronic health conditions. As such, the number of prescription drugs taken may increase. Of all the drug groups available, one group that has been researched with regard to dementia risk is **benzodiazepines**. These drugs are commonly prescribed for anxiety, stress and sleep disorders. However, they may also have a place in the treatment of various other conditions. Benzodiazepines work by interacting with neurotransmitters which transmit messages between brain cells. The action of these drugs is to reduce the excitability of these cells, which results in a calming effect.

A recent study demonstrated that in a 10-year follow-up period, the combination of these agents potentially increases the risk of dementia (Tseng et al., 2019). It was also suggested that taking a shorter-acting drug has a greater risk of dementia than a long-acting drug. However, the mechanisms which increase the risk for dementia in people taking these drugs remains unclear.

Many older individuals also take anti-hypertensive drugs to control blood pressure. While there is currently no evidence to suggest that a specific drug class is more effective than others in lowering the risk of dementia, the lowering of blood pressure may reduce the risk for dementia (Ding et al., 2020).

A large proportion of the population are prescribed drugs such as angiotensin-converting enzyme inhibitors (ACE), diuretics, Beta-blockers, and angiotensin receptor blockers (ARB) for hypertension. A recent network meta-analysis compared antihypertensive drugs with respect to the incidence of dementia and cognitive function, demonstrating that all antihypertensive drugs may, to some extent, be cognitively protective; in particular, ARB's showed significant benefits to cognitive functioning compared with placebos (Marpillat et al., 2013). However, further studies need to be conducted to substantiate these results.

High levels of midlife total cholesterol have been associated with compromised late-life episodic memory, slower psychomotor speed (Solomon et al., 2009; Fratiglioni et al., 2010; Ma et al., 2017) and a higher risk of Alzheimer's disease. However, a number of studies indicate that statin medications which are often prescribed to treat high cholesterol, may themselves impact adversely on cognition, possibly through side effects including increased physical and mental fatigue (Gnjidic et al., 2015; Chatterjee et al., 2015.).

A relatively large proportion of the older population are also taking antidepressant medications. There is evidence to suggest that antidepressants have a significant positive effect on psychomotor speed and delayed memory recall (Rosenblat et al., 2016). Further clinical research needs to be conducted within this area to assess the cognitive effectiveness of antidepressants and whether they can offset the negative impact of depression on cognition and brain health.

Many older adults are also often prescribed non-steroidal anti-inflammatory drugs (NSAID's) such as ibuprofen. There is mixed evidence overall concerning whether these medications increase your risk for dementia. This is mainly related to the side effects of particular drugs. For instance, ibuprofen is often prescribed due to its lesser effects on the stomach and on the kidneys and so may be associated with a decreased risk for dementia compared with others which have greater effects on these systems. However, it is also noted that some NSAID's can sometimes increase blood pressure, which may have implications for cognitive function. However, it is important to acknowledge that it may not be the medications which increase the risk for cognitive decline. Instead, it may be the pain the individual is experiencing which has led them to take these medications (Whitlock, 2017).

While the mechanisms behind any increased risk associated with taking medication is unclear, it may be related in part to neuronal damage associated with the health conditions that the medication is treating, rather than the medication itself. Therefore, all medications used within an ageing population need to have further clinical investigations made to determine the impact on cognitive decline and/or dementia.

CHAPTER 6:
How do you feed your Brain?

As a functional organ, the brain can be considered to be the most sophisticated 'computer' ever designed which has been unable to be replicated, even with advancements in technology. Therefore, it is essential to understand what the brain needs to survive to live a long and healthy life. In this section, we will explore these requirements and start to establish the essence of brain health.

In essence, your brain is a massive consumer of the body's resources. These resources are obtained through the food that we consume. Over time, our understanding of food, the way food is grown (e.g. soil nutrients) and the types of foods available has changed drastically. As such, we now have a greater understanding and control over what contributes to a good healthy diet and what contributes to a poor diet. Moreover, scientists have come to understand that certain nutrients and other key chemical compounds contained within the food that we eat is what is essential for human brain function. Consider this: if you need your petrol-driven car to function correctly, you do not fill it with diesel fuel. It is the same with our brain; it requires specific essential nutrients to be able to function properly. For instance, the development and repair of neural tissue within the brain is dependent on the proper intake of essential structural nutrients, minerals, and vitamins. Deficiencies in some of these vitamins can lead to impaired cognitive function due to neurological or nerve fibre complications.

Throughout different stages in an individual's life, it is thought that the brain has different energy demands. Therefore, nutritional requirements also change, which is important for optimal functioning (Le Coutre et al., 2013). For instance, one recent finding suggests that by improving the diet of older people, the onset or progression of age-related cognitive decline processes may be delayed (Deary et al., 2009).

The importance of a healthy diet for a healthy brain has led many researchers to suggest that a diet rich in B-vitamins, antioxidants and omega-3's are required for mental fitness.

The B Vitamins

A lack of basic B vitamins (folic acid, B6 and B12) in the diet is proposed to impact the rate of brain atrophy associated with mild cognitive impairment and with healthy ageing (Mathers, 2013). The B-complex vitamins, including B1-thiamine, B2-riboflavin, B3-niacin, B5-pantothenate, B6, biotin, B9-folate and B12-cobalamin, are obtained from the diet and are required for the production of neurotransmitters, and as such, have a strong role to play in brain function and modulation of mood.

In adults, low B-vitamin status (particularly folate and vitamins B6 and B12) has been associated with internalising behavioural problems such as depression (Sanchez-Villegas et al., 2009; Skarupski et al., 2010). This is related to the role of vitamin B6 in synthesising neurotransmitters, including serotonin, epinephrine, norepinephrine and gamma-aminobutyric acid (Gomez-Pinilla, 2008). Evidence suggests that vitamin supplementation with B6 (Wyatt et al., 1999) and folate may improve depressive symptoms, as folate has been reported to increase the efficacy of antidepressants or other psychiatric medications (Coppen & Bailey, 2000).

The B vitamins have also been identified as regulators of homocysteine levels which is considered to be a risk factor associated with cognitive decline. Normally, vitamin B12, B6, and folic acid break down homocysteine and change it into other substances your body needs (Ordovas, 2008). Therefore, if deficient in B vitamins, homocysteine levels may build up, which may lead to potential long-term damage in the brain.

Antioxidants

Oxidative stress has been implicated in age-related cognitive decline. It was suggested by Van Dyke and Sano (2007) that dietary antioxidants such as vitamin E, beta-carotene and flavonoids which are found in fruit and vegetables, may have a protective effect against oxidative damage to the brain by enhancing the antioxidant defences. In addition to this work, it has been suggested that plant polyphenols interact with ageing neurons in the brain, increasing the neurons' capacity to maintain effective and proper functioning during the ageing process (Gomez-Pinilla, 2008; Van Dyk & Sano, 2007). Polyphenol compounds, such as flavonoids, phenolic acids and tannins, have been discovered in a range of plant-based food sources (e.g. legumes, fruit, vegetables, herbal extracts, spices, tea and cocoa). Specifically, (poly)phenols have been associated with a number of health benefits, including the modulation of inflammation, reductions in risks of cardiovascular disease, anti-cancer and protection against oxidative stress within the body and brain (Ammar et al., 2020).

Omega-3's

It has been proposed that a high intake of seafood and other sources of long-chain omega-3 polyunsaturated fats (LC-n3-FA) may have long-term beneficial effects on cognitive function (Fotuhi et al., 2009; Witte et al., 2013). The addition of regular fish (which is a rich source of omega-3's) to one's diet has also been shown to maintain grey matter volumes in the hippocampus and other areas within the brain (Raji et al., 2014). In a recent study, it was reported that high-DHA (omega 3) supplementation produced similar improvements in cognitive function observed with aerobic exercise. This is an interesting outcome as supplementation may be able to reduce the negative effects of low physical activity on cognitive function in an elderly population (Fairbairn et al., 2019).

Dietary patterns

The nutritional intake of an individual is a complex interaction of macro (proteins, fats and carbohydrates) and micronutrients (vitamins and minerals). As a result of these interactions, recent research has focused on the effect of **dietary patterns** as they may be more inclusive and representative of what individuals typically eat. As such, dietary patterns can be described as a particular type of diet that you may normally adhere to.

To date, a form of the **Mediterranean diet** - rich in fruits and vegetables, legumes, and low in meat, poultry and dairy products has been considered a potential way to maximise cognitive ability in old age. It is proposed by Warnberg et al. (2009) that a healthy diet such as this has a dual effect on reducing the effects of inflammation and amelioration of a neurodegenerative disorder. High consumption of fruit and vegetables or a diet that is full of antioxidants, serum carotenoids, vitamins, fibre and magnesium can be extremely beneficial in reducing C reactive protein (CRP) levels - a sensitive measure of inflammation in the body (Ajani et al., 2004; Wärnberg et al., 2009a).

In contrast, a diet high in refined sugar, cholesterol, and trans-fats might be associated with a poor diet and poorer cognitive outcomes in older age (Ordovas, 2008). For instance, a poor diet is associated with increased mental health and behavioural problems (Herbison et al., 2012). As such, this may, in part, explain the observation that the lifetime prevalence of mental health disorders in many Western populations is approaching 50% (World Health Organisation [WHO], 2000: https://www.who.int/whr/2000/en/).

How does the food I eat cause cognitive changes?

It is considered that the role of nutrition on cognitive performance is complex and multifactorial. However, the long-term effects of nutrition on cognition may be considered to fall into the following groups:

- Glucose: food that provides energy for the brain
- Lipids and amino acids: the building blocks and
- Micronutrients (iron, zinc, B Vitamins, iodine): the main source of bio-or psychoactive molecules which can exert multiple relevant brain actions (LeCoutre & Schmitt., 2008, Gomez-Pinilla., 2008).

Our overall diet can affect other risk factors such as inflammation and oxidation within the body and brain. Diets that are low in energy and that act to reduce oxidative stress may be protective against cognitive decline (Budge et al.,

2000). Conversely, a diet that is high in energy and acts to increase oxidative stress may be considered a risk factor for impaired cognitive functioning (Butterfield et al., 2002).

Diet can also instigate changes in various neurobiological markers in the blood. These can cross the blood-brain barrier and have an impact on cognitive function. For instance, when someone is fasting or suffering from strict food restrictions, there is a reduction in **Brain-Derived Neurotrophic Factor (BDNF)** levels. BDNF plays a role in regulating glucose metabolism, which can impact how much energy the brain receives. Additionally, low levels of BDNF may trigger binge episodes and weight gain in individuals and have been associated with a high risk of eating disorders such as anorexia nervosa and bulimia nervosa and have a role in food intake regulation.

The gut microbiota (microorganisms in your gut that help control digestion and benefit your immune system) play an essential role in the functioning of many organs in the body including the brain. Despite our current limited knowledge of specific mechanisms, dietary and microbial modulation show promise as potential strategies to tackle some neurodegenerative and neurological diseases. A more comprehensive understanding of gut microbial ecology, metabolism, and signalling networks within our body may lead to a new generation of microbiome-targeted strategies, both for disease treatment and prevention. (Parker et al., 2020).

Summary

Dietary factors have been considered a powerful influence on brain function on a daily basis. A diet rich in saturated fats (such as fatty meats, trans fats from fast food, excess dairy) decreases learning and memory and increases metabolic distress. The effects of a poor diet, however, can be overcome by the effects of exercise. It has been suggested that diet (one that is high in fruit and vegetables) and exercise can assist the brain in coping with several types of insults and ultimately benefit brain function over time (Pinilla, 2006).

Therefore, what we eat or what we choose not to eat may have an important impact on our cognitive ability and mental performance over our lifetime (Sizonenko et al., 2013).

CHAPTER 7:
When is the time to take action?

From what we have already discussed, it is clear that changes occurring in the brain are lifelong, and therefore, the time to take action is now! It is generally accepted that the brain is fully developed by the age of 25, and with declines in abilities and changes in brain structures occurring from then on, it is never really too late to start engaging in activities which may help to preserve brain function.

As touched on previously, the brain's ability to resist damage is called **cognitive reserve**; this is the sum of all of the positive things done throughout life to help the brain (e.g. good diet, exercise, mental stimulation etc.) and the negative things which may impact cognitive function (e.g. exposure to environmental toxins, alcohol and drug abuse etc.). So, the more positive behaviours that you engage in, the better your cognitive reserve is likely to be and the better your brain will be able to fight or recover from damage.

Given that most of the changes associated with dementia and cognitive decline occur in mid-life, the earlier you establish and maintain a higher cognitive reserve, the better as you can fight damage earlier. This is supported by research which suggests that those with a higher cognitive reserve are less likely to experience cognitive decline and are at a lesser risk for dementia (Blennow et al., 2006; Buckner, 2004; Prince et al., 2014). However, engaging in positive activities for the brain later in life can also contribute to your cognitive reserve, which may allow you to fight damage due to late-onset dementia and slow the rate of age-related decline.

Physical activity

Research suggests that exercise and physical activity can have positive effects no matter the life stage. Specifically mid-life exercise has been associated with a reduction in the risk of dementia with some studies suggesting that cognitive benefits can occur within a matter of a few months, even for those who have not been previously active (Farrow et al., 2013). Research also suggests that those with MCI or dementia may experience cognitive benefits following exercise. For instance, the findings of a meta-analysis which looked at the results of 18 intervention studies, found that exercise programs can enhance cognitive function in people with MCI and dementia (Heyn et al., 2004).

Diet

It is no secret that maintaining an unhealthy diet can lead to a host of health problems including weight gain, increased stress on your heart and lungs, high cholesterol and an increased risk for diabetes. The longer you continue to consume an unhealthy diet, the more time fatty deposits have to accumulate in your arteries leading to an increased risk for clots and, thus, stroke. You may also continue to gain weight which can put even more pressure on your body and organs, making it harder to lose weight. Therefore, maintaining a healthy diet from a young age can reduce cardiovascular risks, which can lead to stress and inflammation, thereby affecting the brain. It also allows for an increased opportunity for your brain to receive valuable vitamins and nutrients, which can promote neuronal growth and promote cognitive reserve.

While it is difficult to study whether changes to particular dietary patterns at particular ages can positively impact risk reduction for dementia and cognitive decline, studies investigating the individual effects of increasing intakes of antioxidants, vitamins and nutrients have found some beneficial effects. Given there is evidence that adherence to dietary patterns such as the Mediterranean diet (which include foods which are rich sources of these) is associated with a decreased risk for cognitive decline and dementia, it makes sense to assume that the earlier you begin eating healthily, the better off your brain will be.

Smoking

As we discussed in Chapter 4, the risk for cognitive decline and dementia can be reduced by quitting smoking. However, research suggests that this risk reduction may depend on when you quit. Specifically, it has been found that those who quit nine years ago or more had the same risk for dementia as those who had never smoked. In comparison, the risk for those who had recently quit (within the last 9 years) was only slightly reduced compared to current smokers (Deal et al., 2020). Similarly, a meta-analysis of studies reported that former smokers had no higher risk for developing dementia compared to those who had never smoked. However, they did have an increased risk for early cognitive decline, although this risk was still lower than that of current smokers (Anstey et al., 2007). This suggests that the longer your body has to enjoy the benefits associated with quitting such as increased blood flow and less stress on your heart, the more likely your brain is to recover and maintain cognitive function.

Summary

It is generally accepted that your overall risk for cognitive decline and dementia is a combination of non-modifiable risk factors as well as modifiable risk factors. As such, one does not simply develop dementia due to age; rather, it may be thought of as having developed over the course of many years, partly due to lifestyle choices. While you may not be able to control your age and genetics, you can certainly control your physical activity and what you eat and as demonstrated, these factors may assist in reducing your risk. While it is assumed that following a healthy lifestyle from a young age is the best approach, research supports that there are benefits to making changes in your mid-life and even into old age. Even small changes can have big effects on your brain health - so the time to act is now.

Change is no easy feat, and having a strong support network can assist you. Talking to your friends and family about the changes you would like to make or committing to making the changes together may help you avoid relapses in your behaviour. We also recommend discussing your lifestyle changes with your doctor to ensure that they are safe and manageable for you. Your doctor may also be able to provide direct support or a referral to other services which can support you further in your journey to good brain health.

CHAPTER 8:
What is the recipe for a Healthy Brain?

In chapters 1 and 2, we provided an overview of the structural and cognitive changes that may be experienced during normal ageing and dementia. In chapter 3, we described the different types of dementia and explained how they differ in terms of the damage that occurs. In chapter 4, we provided an overview of the current evidence regarding various lifestyle factors and the impact they can have on your brain and cognitive function. From there, we addressed some common myths associated with ageing and the development of dementia. Following this, we included a closer look at how what we eat can influence brain development and cognitive ageing. Although it appears that the earlier positive changes are enforced, the better, we provided some evidence that suggests that even changes later in life can be beneficial. Now comes time to put all of this together into a 'recipe' of sorts.

Let's summarise the key points of this book:

- Brain ageing across a lifetime can be considered as the progressive and gradual accumulation of potential detrimental changes in brain cellular structure and function. As such, subtle brain changes that occur earlier in life may indicate an increased risk for brain disease later in life.

- A large number of cognitive changes occurring at once within the brain may result in 'cognitive decline'. Cognitive decline is not the same in every individual, and will vary depending on one's lifestyle choices, ethnicity and genome.

- Most of the changes in the brain that are associated with dementia and cognitive decline occur in mid-life. The earlier you establish and maintain a higher cognitive reserve the better, as you can fight damage earlier.

- The brain can produce new cells and as such, it is 'neuroprotective'. The amount of damage and impact to function may be minimised by modifying lifestyle factors such as diet and behavioural modifications.

- Lifestyle changes are potentially an effective, non-pharmacological intervention that may reduce the effects of ageing on the brain. Two supported lifestyle changes include exercise and diet.

- A high consumption of fruit and vegetables and nuts or a diet full of antioxidants, serum carotenoids, vitamins, fibre, and magnesium are extremely beneficial in reducing inflammatory levels in the brain and modulating mood and maintaining vascular health.

- A Western diet and a sedentary lifestyle impact general health, including increasing the rate of obesity, high blood pressure, high levels of cholesterol and insulin resistance. This may also lead to the development of other health conditions which can contribute to the risk of dementia and cognitive decline.

- Most types of exercise have been shown to have a

beneficial effect on brain function.

So overall, according to this evidence, a well-constructed recipe for dying with a healthy brain might look a little something like this:

Step 1. Optimise your body mass index (BMI):

This is a measurement used for both men and women, providing an estimate of how healthy your weight is in accordance with your height. To calculate your BMI, you divide your weight in kilograms by your height in centimetres squared.

If your BMI is…

- Under 18.5 – you are considered to be underweight.
- 18.5 to 24.9 – you are considered to be within a healthy weight range.
- 25.0 to 29.9 – you are considered to be overweight.
- Over 30 – you are considered to be obese.

However, it is important to note that this is not an accurate measure for all people as it does not take into consideration muscle mass. For example, bodybuilders typically have a high BMI- but this does not necessarily mean that they are unhealthy. Irrespective of this, it remains a good starting point for predicting weight-related issues such as heart problems, cholesterol and diabetes.

Step 2. Ensure a healthy Hip to Waist Ratio (WHR):

WHR measures the ratio of your waist circumference to your hip circumference, determining how much fat is stored on your waist, hips, and buttocks. This is calculated as waist measurement divided by hip measurement (W ÷ H).

This is important because where you carry your weight can have different risks to your health. For example, people who have more weight around their midsections are at higher risk for heart disease, type 2 diabetes, stroke, and premature death, than people who carry their weight in their hips and thighs. Importantly, you can have a healthy BMI and still have excess fat around your midsection, meaning you could still be at risk of developing certain diseases. Below is a guide of where you should be - ideally, we want to aim for low-moderate risk.

Health Risk	Women	Men
Low	0.8 or lower	0.95 or lower
Moderate	0.81-0.85	0.96-0.99
High	0.86	or higher

Step 3. Quit/ reduce smoking:

Don't smoke - it really is that simple! If you are a smoker, then reducing or quitting are also beneficial. Over time, your risk for cognitive decline can lower to almost the same level as a non-smoker.

Step 4. Keep your alcohol intake within recommended limits:

To reduce your risk of alcohol-related harm, disease or injury, it is recommended that healthy men and women drink no more than 10 standard drinks per week and no more than 4 standard drinks on any one day (refer to Department of Health (2020). How much alcohol is safe to drink? https://www.health.gov.au/health-topics/alcohol/about-alcohol/how-much-alcohol-is-safe-to-drink).

Step 5. Optimise your blood pressure:

A normal reading for blood pressure is considered to fall between 90/60 mm Hg and 120/80mm Hg in an adult. If you are in the normal range, no medical intervention is needed. However, you should maintain a healthy lifestyle and healthy weight to help prevent hypertension from developing. If your blood pressure is consistently outside of this range, it is recommended that you speak to your doctor for medical management.

Step 6. Manage your cholesterol:

Keep your fasting blood cholesterol below or equal to the recommendations for your country of origin. In general, total cholesterol levels less than 200 milligrams per decilitre (mg/dL) are considered desirable for adults. A reading between 200 and 239 mg/dL is considered borderline high, and a reading of 240 mg/dL and above is considered high. For LDL cholesterol, levels should be less than 100 mg/dL. If your levels are consistently outside this range, this may indicate issues with your diet or a medical condition. It is recommended that you have your cholesterol tested at least twice a year by your doctor and discuss ways in which you can reduce or maintain healthy levels.

Step 7. Maintain social interactions with your friends and family:

Interacting with others promotes a sense of safety, belonging and security. It allows you to confide in others and let them confide in you. This can lighten your mood and make you feel happier. It can also help you maintain adaptive coping strategies during stressful times, which can lower your risk for some mental disorders. Research also suggests that social interaction is good for your brain health and may lower your risk for dementia.

Step 8. Reduce your dependency on a typical Western Diet:

The Western diet, often characterized by excessive intakes of simple, highly refined sugars and refined oils high in saturated fats, can lead to numerous harmful health implications, resulting in an epidemic of diet-related diseases. Reducing large portions of fatty meats, reducing your salt intake and increasing your portions of fruit and vegetables may assist with this.

Discussing your dietary intake with a qualified professional such as a dietitian may assist you in optimising your diet with consideration of any special dietary needs you have as well as medical conditions and medications.

Step 9. Consider a Mediterranean Style Diet instead:

This is, to date, the world's healthiest diet and is abundant in fruits, vegetables, whole grains, legumes and olive oil. It also features fish and poultry - lean sources of protein over red meat. Red wine is consumed regularly but in moderate amounts (125ml/day). This form of diet is associated with low levels of inflammation which is beneficial for your brain and your overall wellbeing. It is balanced and may assist you to lose and maintain weight.

Step 10. Maintain Exercise:

Regular exercise can have a profoundly positive impact on depression, anxiety, ADHD, and more. It relieves stress, improves memory, helps you sleep better, and boosts your overall mood. For example, even a short burst of 10 minutes' brisk walking increases mental alertness, energy and mood. Further, participation in regular physical activity can increase our self-esteem and can reduce stress and anxiety. Recommendations include at least 20-30 min every day of a variety of physical activities such as walking, riding a bike, gardening and swimming.

As stated earlier, please discuss any changes to exercise or physical activity with your doctor or an exercise physiologist. They will be able to assist you in progressing safely. They can also provide individualised exercises that take into account physical limitations and medical history.

Step 11. Train your Brain:

Brain games may help sharpen your thinking skills that tend to wane with age, such as processing speed, planning skills, reaction time, decision making, and short-term memory. Engaging in activities which are educational such as learning a language or playing music, can keep activities fun and pleasant.

As previously stated, there are also a number of non-modifiable factors which contribute to your risk for cognitive decline. While there is no guarantee that following these recommendations will keep you dementia-free, you can rest assured that you are promoting the best environment and lifestyle for your brain and your general health.

Although recommendations suggest that it is ideal to start this process during mid-life, making changes at any age will promote positive changes and promote cognitive reserve in your brain.

If you take on the research and the understanding of what this represents, there is a very good chance, according to the research that we have presented, that you will have a recipe for a healthy brain and potentially die with a healthy brain.

References for all Chapters

References Chapter 1

Anderson, M. F., Åberg, M. A. I., Nilsson, M., & Eriksson, P. S. (2002). Insulin-like growth factor-I and neurogenesis in the adult mammalian brain. *Developmental Brain Research, 134*(1-2), 115-122. doi:10.1016/s0165-3806(02)00277-8

Behar, T. N., Schaffner, A. E., Scott, C. A., O'Connell, C., & Barker, J. L. (1998). Differential response of cortical plate and ventricular zone cells to GABA as a migration stimulus. *Journal of Neuroscience*, 18(16), 6378-6387.

Burke, S. N., & Barnes, C. A. (2006). Neural plasticity in the ageing brain. *Nature Reviews Neuroscience,* 7(1), 30-40. doi:10.1038/nrn1809

Chen, G. C., Yang, J., Eggersdorfer, M., Zhang, W. G., & Qin, L. Q. (2016). N-3 long-chain polyunsaturated fatty acids and risk of all-cause mortality among general populations: a meta-analysis. *Scientific Reports, 6.* doi:10.1038/srep28165

Colombo, B., Antonietti, A., & Daneau, B. (2018). The Relationships Between Cognitive Reserve and Creativity. A Study on American Aging Population. *Frontiers in Psychology,* 9. doi:10.3389/fpsyg.2018.00764

Coutre, J. L., & Schmitt, J. A. J. (2008). Food ingredients and cognitive performance. *Current Opinion in Clinical Nutrition and Metabolic Care,* 11(6), 706-710. doi:10.1097/MCO.0b013e32831394a5

Fernandes, J., Arida, R. M., & Gomez-Pinilla, F. (2017). Physical exercise as an epigenetic modulator of brain plasticity and cognition. *Neuroscience and Biobehavioral Reviews,* 80, 443-456. doi:10.1016/j.neubiorev.2017.06.012

Fratiglioni, L., Mangialasche, F., & Qiu, C. (2010). Brain aging: lessons from community studies. *Nutrition Reviews, 68*(12), S119-S127. doi:10.1111/j.1753-4887.2010.00353.x

Gesch, C. B., Hammond, S. M., Hampson, S. E., Eves, A., & Crowder, M. J. (2002). Influence of supplementary vitamins, minerals and essential fatty acids on the antisocial behaviour of young adult prisoners. Randomised, placebo-controlled trial. *British Journal of Psychiatry, 181*(JULY), 22-28. doi:10.1192/bjp.181.1.22

Global Nutrition. (2018). *Current Developments in Nutrition,* 2(11). doi:10.1093/cdn/nzy039

Huizinga, W., Poot, D. H. J., Vernooij, M. W., Roshchupkin, G. V., Bron, E. E., Ikram, M. A., . . . Alzheimers Dis, N. (2018). A spatio-temporal reference model of the aging brain. *Neuroimage, 169,* 11-22. doi:10.1016/j.neuroimage.2017.10.040

Kennedy, D. O. (2016). B Vitamins and the Brain: Mechanisms, Dose and Efficacy-A Review. *Nutrients, 8*(2). doi:10.1002/HUP.2236; 10.3390/nu8020068

Kennedy, G., Hardman, R., Macpherson, H., Meyer, D., Scholey, A., & Pipingas, A. (2016). The LIILAC Trial: Effects of Aerobic Exercise and Mediterranean Diet on Cognition in Cognitively Healthy Older People Living Independently Within Aged Care Facilities. *Journal of Aging and Physical Activity, 24,* S19-S20.

Kirkwood, T. B. L. (2008). A systematic look at an old problem. *Nature, 451*(7179), 644-647. doi:10.1038/451644a

Mattson, M. P., Chan, S. L., & Duan, W. (2002). Modification of brain aging and neurodegenerative disorders by genes, diet, and behavior. *Physiological Reviews, 82*(3), 637-672.

Nilsson, J., & Lovden, M. (2018). Naming is not explaining: future directions for the 'cognitive reserve' and 'brain maintenance' theories. *Alzheimer's Research & Therapy, 10.* doi:10.1186/s13195-018-0365-z

Ordovas. (2008). *Nutrition and cognitive health.* London: The Government Office of science.

Park, D. C., & Reuter-Lorenz, P. (2009). The Adaptive Brain: Aging and Neurocognitive Scaffolding *Annual Review of Psychology* (Vol. 60, pp. 173-196).

Peters. (2006). Ageing and the brain. *Post Graduate Medical Journal, 82,* 84-88. doi:10.1136/pgmj.2005.036665

Reisberg, B., Franssen, E. H., Hasan, S. M., Monteiro, I., Boksay, I., Souren, L. E. M., . . . Kluger, A. (1999). Retrogenesis: clinical, physiologic, and pathologic mechanisms in brain aging, Alzheimer's and other dementing processes. *European Archives of Psychiatry and Clinical Neuroscience, 249,* 28-36.

Scheller, E., Schumacher, L. V., Peter, J., Lahr, J., Wehrle, J., Kaller, C. P., . . . Kloppel, S. (2018). Brain Aging and APOE epsilon 4 Interact to Reveal Potential Neuronal Compensation in Healthy Older Adults. *Frontiers in Aging Neuroscience, 10.* doi:10.3389/fnagi.2018.00074

Uauy, R., & Dangour, A. D. (2006). Nutrition in brain development and aging: Role of essential fatty acids. *Nutrition Reviews, 64*(5), S24-S33. doi:10.1301/nr.2006.may.S24-S33

Van Dyk, K., & Sano, M. (2007). The impact of nutrition on cognition in the elderly. *Neurochemical Research, 32*(4-5), 893-904. doi:10.1007/s11064-006-9241-5

Yankner, B. A., Lu, T., & Loerch, P. (2008). The aging brain *Annual Review of Pathology-Mechanisms of Disease* (Vol. 3, pp. 41-66).

References Chapter 2

Australian Institute of Health and Welfare. (2012). *Dementia in Australia.*

Cabeza, R., Daselaar, S. M., Dolcos, F., Prince, S. E., Budde, M., & Nyberg, L. (2004). Task-independent and task-specific age effects on brain activity during working memory, visual attention and episodic retrieval. *Cerebral Cortex, 14*(4), 364-375. doi:10.1093/cercor/bhg133

Chan, R. C. K., Shum, D., Toulopoulou, T., & Chen, E. Y. H. (2008). Assessment of executive functions: Review of instruments and identification of critical issues. *Archives of Clinical Neuropsychology, 23*(2), 201-216. doi:10.1016/j.acn.2007.08.010

Christensen, H. (2001). What cognitive changes can be expected with normal ageing? *Australian and New Zealand Journal of Psychiatry, 35*(6), 768-775. doi:10.1046/j.1440-1614.2001.00966.x

Christensen .H., K. R. (2003). The Neurology and Neuropsychology of Ageing. 75-97.

Deary, I. J., Corley, J., Gow, A. J., Harris, S. E., Houlihan, L. M., Marioni, R. E., . . . Starr, J. M. (2009). *Age-associated cognitive decline. z*(1), 135-152. doi:10.1093/bmb/ldp033

Di Paolo T. (1994). Modulation of brain dopamine transmission by sex steroids. Rev Neurosci. 1994 Jan-Mar;5(1):27-41. doi: 10.1515/revneuro.1994.5.1.27. PMID: 8019704

Greenwood, & Parasurman. (2010). Neuronal and cognitive plasticity: neurocognitive framework for ameliorating cognitive aging. *Frontiers in Aging Neurosciences, 2*(150), 1-14.

Greenwood, P. M. (2007). Functional Plasticity in Cognitive Aging: Review and Hypothesis. *Neuropsychology, 21*(6), 657-673. doi:10.1037/0894-4105.21.6.657

Gunstad, J., Paul, R. H., Brickman, A. M., Cohen, R. A., Arns, M., Roe, D., . . . Gordon, E. (2006). Patterns of cognitive performance in middle-aged and older adults: A cluster analytic examination. *Journal of Geriatric Psychiatry and Neurology, 19*(2), 59-64. doi:10.1177/0891988705284738

Jagger, C., Gillies, C., Moscone, F., & Team, E. (2008). Inequalities in healthy life years in the 25 countries of the European Union in 2005: a cross-national meta-regression analysis (vol 372, pg 2124, 2008). *Lancet, 372*(9656), 2114-2114.

Loewenstein, D. A., Acevedo, A., Czaja, S. J., & Duara, R. (2004). Cognitive rehabilitation of mildly impaired Alzheimer disease Patients on cholinesterase inhibitors. *American Journal of Geriatric Psychiatry, 12*(4), 395-402. doi:10.1176/appi.ajgp.12.4.395

McKenzie, K., Metcalfe, D., & Murray, G. (2018). A review of measures used in the screening, assessment and diagnosis of dementia in people with an intellectual disability. *Journal of Applied Research in Intellectual Disabilities, 31*(5), 725-742. doi:10.1111/jar.12441

Mukadam, N., Sommerlad, A., Huntley, J., & Livingston, G. (2019). Potential for dementia prevention in Latin America and Africa based on population-attributable fraction estimates. *Lancet Global Health, 7*(10), E1325-E1325. doi:10.1016/s2214-109x(19)30331-6

Park, D. C., & Reuter-Lorenz, P. (2009). The Adaptive Brain: Aging and Neurocognitive Scaffolding *Annual Review of Psychology* (Vol. 60, pp. 173-196).

Pipingas, A., Harris, E., Tournier, E., King, R., Kras, M., & Stough, C. K. (2010). ASSESSING THE EFFICACY OF NUTRACEUTICAL INTERVENTIONS ON COGNITIVE FUNCTIONING IN THE ELDERLY. *Current Topics in Nutraceutical Research, 8*(2-3), 79-87.

Reynolds, C. A., Gatz, M., & Pedersen, N. L. (2002). Individual variation for cognitive decline: Quantitative methods for describing patterns of change. *Psychology and Aging, 17*(2), 271-287. doi:10.1037//0882-7974.17.2.271

Salthouse, T. A. (2012a). Are individual differences in rates of aging greater at older ages? *Neurobiology of Aging, 33*(10), 2373-2381. doi:10.1016/j.neurobiolaging.2011.10.018

Salthouse, T. A. (2012b). Does the Level at Which Cognitive Change Occurs Change With Age? *Psychological Science, 23*(1), 18-23. doi:10.1177/0956797611421615

Sourdet, S., Rouge-Bugat, M. E., Vellas, B., & Forette, F. (2012). Frailty and aging. *Journal of Nutrition Health & Aging, 16*(4), 283-284. doi:10.1007/s12603-012-0040-1

References Chapter 3

Australian Institute of Health and Welfare. (2012). *Dementia in Australia.*

Blennow, K., de Leon, M. J., & Zetterberg, H. (2006). Alzheimer's disease. *The Lancet, 368*(9533), 387-403. doi:http://dx.doi.org/10.1016/S0140-6736(06)69113-7

Boot, B. P., McDade, E. M., McGinnis, S. M., & Boeve, B. F. (2013). Treatment of dementia with lewy bodies. *Current treatment options in neurology, 15*(6), 738-764. doi:10.1007/s11940-013-0261-6

Brown, L., Hansnata, E., & La, H. A. (2017). *Economic cost of Dementia in Australia.* https://www.dementia.org.au/sites/default/files/NATIONAL/documents/The-economic-cost-of-dementia-in-Australia-2016-to-2056.pdf

Buckner, R. L. (2004). Memory and Executive Function in Aging and AD: Multiple Factors that Cause Decline and Reserve Factors that Compensate. *Neuron, 44*(1), 195-208. doi:http://dx.doi.org/10.1016/j.neuron.2004.09.006

Dementia Australia. (2000). *Frontotemporal dementia help sheet.* https://www.dementia.org.au/resources/help-sheets

Dementia Australia. (2016). Younger onset dementia help sheet 21.

Economics, A. (2009). *Keeping Dementia front of mind: incidence and prevalence 2009-2050.* https://researchers.mq.edu.au/en/publications/keeping-dementia-front-of-mind-incidence-and-prevalence-2009-2050

Heggie, M., Morgan, D., Crossley, M., Kirk, A., Wong, P., Karunanayake, C., & Beever, R. (2012). Quality of life in early dementia: Comparison of rural patient and caregiver ratings at baseline and one year. *Dementia, 11*(4), 521-541.

Libon, D. J., Scanlon, M., Swenson, R., Branch Coslet, H. J. J. o. G. P., & Neurology. (1990). Binswanger's disease: some neuropsychological considerations. 3(1), 31-40.

Prince, M., Albanese, E., Guerchet, M., & Prina, M. (2014). *World Alzheimer Report 2014. Dementia and risk reduction: an analysis of protective and modifiable factors.* https://www.alzint.org/u/WorldAlzheimerReport2014.pdf

References Chapter 4

The National Health and Medical Research Council (NHMRC), (2014). *Proposal for national project to reduce or delay cognitive decline and dementia.* https://www.nhmrc.gov.au › file › downloadPDF

Ahlskog, J. E., Geda, Y. E., Graff-Radford, N. R., & Petersen, R. C. (2011). Physical exercise as a preventive or disease-modifying treatment of dementia and brain aging. *Mayo Clinic Proceedings, 86*(9), 876-884. doi:10.4065/mcp.2011.025

Anderson-Hanley, C., Nimon, J. P., & Westen, S. C. (2010). Cognitive health benefits of strengthening exercise for community-dwelling older adults. *Journal of Clinical and Experimental Neuropsychology, 32*(9), 996-1001.

Arab, L., & Sabbagh, M. N. (2010). Are certain lifestyle habits associated with lower Alzheimer's disease risk? *Journal of Alzheimer's Disease, 20*(3), 785-794.

Barnes, D. E., & Yaffe, K. (2011). The projected effect of risk factor reduction on Alzheimer's disease prevalence. *The Lancet Neurology, 10*(9), 819-828.

Best, J. R., Chiu, B. K., Hsu, C. L., Nagamatsu, L. S., & Liu-Ambrose, T. (2015). Long-Term Effects of Resistance Exercise Training on Cognition and Brain Volume in Older Women: Results from a Randomized Controlled Trial. *Journal of the International Neuropsychological Society, 21*(10), 745-756.

Bolandzadeh, N., Tam, R., Handy, T. C., Nagamatsu, L. S., Hsu, C. L., Davis, J. C., . . . Liu-Ambrose, T. (2015). Resistance Training and White Matter Lesion Progression in Older Women: Exploratory Analysis of a 12-Month Randomized Controlled Trial. *Journal of the American Geriatrics Society, 63*(10), 2052-2060. doi:10.1111/jgs.13644

Bottaccioli, A. G., Bottaccioli, F., & Minelli, A. (2019). Stress and the psyche-brain-immune network in psychiatric diseases based on psychoneuroendocrineimmunology: a concise review. *Annals of the New York Academy of Sciences, 1437*(1), 31-42. doi:10.1111/nyas.13728

- Braak, H., Del Tredici, K., Schultz, C., & Braak, E. (2000). Vulnerability of select neuronal types to Alzheimer's disease. In Z. S. Khachaturian & M. M. Mesulam (Eds.), *Alzheimer's Disease: A Compendium of Current Theories* (Vol. 924, pp. 53-61).

- Brown, L., Hansnata, E., & La, H. A. (2017). *Economic cost of Dementia in Australia*. Retrieved from

- Buckner, R. L. (2004). Memory and Executive Function in Aging and AD: Multiple Factors that Cause Decline and Reserve Factors that Compensate. *Neuron, 44*(1), 195-208. doi:http://dx.doi.org/10.1016/j.neuron.2004.09.006

Cassilhas, R. C., Viana, V. A. R., Grassmann, V., Santos, R. T., Santos, R. F., Tufik, S., & Mello, M. T. (2007). The impact of resistance exercise on the cognitive function of the elderly. *Medicine and Science in Sports and Exercise, 39*(8), 1401-1407.

Çınar, N., & Sahiner, T. A. H. (2020). Effects of the online computerized cognitive training program BEYNEX on the cognitive tests of individuals with subjective cognitive impairment and Alzheimer's disease on rivastigmine therapy. *Turkish Journal of Medical Sciences, 50*(1), 231-238. doi:10.3906/sag-1905-244

Colcombe, S., & Kramer, A. F. (2003). Fitness effects on the cognitive function of older adults a meta-analytic study. *Psychological science, 14*(2), 125-130.

Cordain, L., Eaton, S. B., Sebastian, A., Mann, N., Lindeberg, S., Watkins, B. A., . . . Brand-Miller, J. (2005). Origins and evolution of the Western diet: health implications for the 21st century. *The American journal of clinical nutrition, 81*(2), 341-354.

Cotman, C. W., & Berchtold, N. C. (2002). Exercise: a behavioral intervention to enhance brain health and plasticity. Trends in neurosciences, 25(6), 295-301.

Cotman, C. W., Berchtold, N. C., & Christie, L.-A. (2007). Exercise builds brain health: key roles of growth factor cascades and inflammation. *Trends in neurosciences, 30*(9), 464-472.

Dalgas, U., Stenager, E., Lund, C., Rasmussen, C., Petersen, T., Sørensen, H., . . . Overgaard, K. (2013). Neural drive increases following resistance training in patients with multiple sclerosis. *Journal of neurology, 260*(7), 1822-1832.

Davenport, M. H., Hogan, D. B., Eskes, G. A., Longman, R. S., & Poulin, M. J. (2012). Cerebrovascular reserve: the link between fitness and cognitive function? *Exercise and sport sciences reviews, 40*(3), 153-158.

de Camargo, A. (2016). The effects of strength training on cognitive performance in elderly women. *Clinical Interventions in Aging, 11,* 749-754.

Deal, J. A., Power, M. C., Palta, P., Alonso, A., Schneider, A. L. C., Perryman, K., . . . Sharrett, A. R. (2020). Relationship of Cigarette Smoking and Time of Quitting with Incident Dementia and Cognitive Decline. *Journal of the American Geriatrics Society, 68*(2), 337-345.

Deslandes, A., Moraes, H., Ferreira, C., Veiga, H., Silveira, H., Mouta, R., . . . Laks, J. (2009). Exercise and mental health: many reasons to move. *Neuropsychobiology, 59*(4), 191-198.

Falck, R. S., Davis, J. C., Best, J. R., Li, L. C., Chan, P. C. Y., Wyrough, A. B., . . . Liu-Ambrose, T. (2018). Buying time: a proof-of-concept randomized controlled trial to improve sleep quality and cognitive function among older adults with mild cognitive impairment. *Trials, 19*(1), 445. doi:10.1186/s13063-018-2837-7

- Fang, W. L., Jiang, M. J., Gu, B. B., Wei, Y. M., Fan, S. N., Liao, W., . . . Liu, J. (2018). Tooth loss as a risk factor for dementia: systematic review and meta-analysis of 21 observational studies. *Bmc Psychiatry, 18.* doi:10.1186/s12888-018-1927-0

- Farrow, M., Ellis, K., Matters, Y. B., & Australia, F. (2013). *Physical Activity for Brain Health and Fighting Dementia.* Retrieved from

Gates, N. J., Valenzuela, M., Sachdev, P. S., Singh, N. A., Baune, B. T., Brodaty, H., . . . Wang, Y. (2011). Study of Mental Activity and Regular Training (SMART) in at risk individuals: A randomised double blind, sham controlled, longitudinal trial. *BMC geriatrics, 11*(1), 19.

Gatz, M., Mortimer, J. A., Fratiglioni, L., Johansson, B., Berg, S., Reynolds, C. A., & Pedersen, N. L. (2006). Potentially modifiable risk factors for dementia in identical twins. *Alzheimer's & Dementia, 2*(2), 110-117.

Heyn, P., Abreu, B. C., & Ottenbacher, K. J. (2004). The effects of exercise training on elderly persons with cognitive impairment and dementia: a meta-analysis. *Archives of Physical Medicine and Rehabilitation, 85*(10), 1694-1704.

Hultsch, D. F., Hertzog, C., Small, B. J., & Dixon, R. A. (1999). Use it or lose it: Engaged lifestyle as a buffer of cognitive decline in aging? *Psychology and Aging, 14*(2), 245-263. doi:10.1037/0882-7974.14.2.245

Ikudome, S., Mori, S., Unenaka, S., Kawanishi, M., Kitamura, T., & Nakamoto, H. (2016). Effect of Long-Term Body-Mass-Based Resistance Exercise on Cognitive Function in Elderly People. *Journal of Applied Gerontology,* 1-15.

Kanoski, S. E., & Davidson, T. L. (2011). Western diet consumption and cognitive impairment: links to hippocampal dysfunction and obesity. *Physiology & behavior, 103*(1), 59-68.

Kiefte-de Jong, J. C., Mathers, J. C., & Franco, O. H. (2014). Nutrition and healthy ageing: the key ingredients. *Proceedings of the Nutrition Society, 73*(02), 249-259.

Kitamura, S., Katayose, Y., Nakazaki, K., Motomura, Y., Oba, K., Katsunuma, R., . . . Mishima, K. (2016). Estimating individual optimal sleep duration and potential sleep debt. *Scientific Reports, 6.* doi:10.1038/srep35812

Knöchel, C., Oertel-Knöchel, V., O'Dwyer, L., Prvulovic, D., Alves, G., Kollmann, B., & Hampel, H. (2012). Cognitive and behavioural effects of physical exercise in psychiatric patients. *Progress in Neurobiology, 96*(1), 46-68. doi:http://dx.doi.org/10.1016/j.pneurobio.2011.11.007

Larson, E. B., & Bruce, R. A. (1987). Health benefits of exercise in an aging society. *Archives of Internal Medicine, 147*(2), 353-356. doi:10.1001/archinte.1987.00370020171058

Laurin, D., Verreault, R., Lindsay, J., MacPherson, K., & Rockwood, K. (2001). Physical activity and risk of cognitive impairment and dementia in elderly persons. *Archives of Neurology, 58*(3), 498-504.

Laurin, D., Verreault, R., Lindsay, J., MacPherson, K., & Rockwood, K. (2001). Risk factors for Alzheimer's disease: A prospective analysis from the Canadian Study of health and ageing. *Archives of neurology, 58*(3), 498-504.

Lautenschlager, N. T., Cox, K., & Cyarto, E. V. (2012). The influence of exercise on brain aging and dementia. *Biochimica et Biophysica Acta (BBA)-Molecular Basis of Disease, 1822*(3), 474-481.

Lim, K. H.-L., Pysklywec, A., Plante, M., & Demers, L. (2019). The effectiveness of Tai Chi for short-term cognitive function improvement in the early stages of dementia in the elderly: a systematic literature review. *Clinical Interventions in Aging, 14*, 827-839. doi:10.2147/CIA.S202055

Liu-Ambrose, T., Nagamatsu, L. S., Graf, P., Beattie, B. L., Ashe, M. C., & Handy, T. C. (2010). Resistance training and executive functions: A 12-month randomized controlled trial. *Archives of Internal Medicine, 170*(2), 170-178.

Liu-Ambrose, T., Nagamatsu, L. S., Voss, M. W., Khan, K. M., & Handy, T. C. (2012). Resistance training and functional plasticity of the aging brain: a 12-month randomized controlled trial. *Neurobiology of aging, 33*(8), 1690-1698.

Manzo-Avalos, S., & Saavedra-Molina, A. (2010). Cellular and mitochondrial effects of alcohol consumption. *International journal of environmental research and public health, 7*(12), 4281-4304. doi:10.3390/ijerph7124281

Matta Mello Portugal, E., Cevada, T., Sobral Monteiro-Junior, R., Teixeira Guimarães, T., da Cruz Rubini, E., Lattari, E., . . . Camaz Deslandes, A. (2013). *Neuroscience of exercise: from neurobiology mechanisms to mental health. Neuropsychobiology, 68*(1), 1-14.

Miotto, E. C., Batista, A. X., Simon, S. S., & Hampstead, B. M. (2018). Neurophysiologic and Cognitive Changes Arising from Cognitive Training Interventions in Persons with Mild Cognitive Impairment: A Systematic Review. *Neural Plasticity, 1-14.* doi:10.1155/2018/7301530

Netz, Y., Wu, M.-J., Becker, B. J., & Tenenbaum, G. (2005). Physical activity and psychological well-being in advanced age: a meta-analysis of intervention studies. *Psychology and Aging, 20*(2), 272.

Ni, H., Li, C., Feng, X., & Cen, J.-N. (2011). Effects of forced running exercise on cognitive function and its relation to zinc homeostasis-related gene expression in rat hippocampus. *Biological Trace Element Research, 142*(3), 704-712. doi:10.1007/s12011-010-8793-z

Okoro, T., Morrison, V., Maddison, P., Lemmey, A., & Andrew, J. (2013). An assessment of the impact of behavioural cognitions on function in patients partaking in a trial of early home-based progressive resistance training after total hip replacement surgery. *Disability & Rehabilitation, 35*(23), 2000-2007.

Ortega, R. M., Requejo, A. M., Andres, P., López-Sobaler, A. M., Quintas, M. E., Redondo, M. R., . . . Rivas, T. (1997). Dietary intake and cognitive function in a group of elderly people. *The American journal of clinical nutrition, 66*(4), 803-809.

Pappas, M. A., & Drigas, A. S. (2019). Computerized Training for Neuroplasticity and Cognitive Improvement. *International Journal of Engineering Pedagogy, 9*(4), 50-62. doi:10.3991/ijep.v9i4.10285

Peters, R., Poulter, R., Warner, J., Beckett, N., Burch, L., & Bulpitt, C. (2008). Smoking, dementia and cognitive decline in the elderly, a systematic review. *BMC geriatrics, 8,* 36. doi:10.1186/1471-2318-8-36

Samieri, C., Okereke, O. I., Devore, E. E., & Grodstein, F. (2013). Long-term adherence to the mediterranean diet is associated with overall cognitive status, but not cognitive decline, in women. *The Journal of nutrition, 143*(4), 493-499.

Sittiprapaporn, P. (2020). Cognitive skills improved by BrainWare SAFARI training program: Electroencephalographic study. *Asian Journal of Medical Sciences, 11*(1), 57-62. doi:10.3126/ajms.v11i1.26526

Siu, M.-Y., & Lee, D. T. F. (2018). Effects of tai chi on cognition and instrumental activities of daily living in community dwelling older people with mild cognitive impairment. *BMC geriatrics, 18*(1), 37-37. doi:10.1186/s12877-018-0720-8

Solfrizzi, V., Panza, F., & Capurso, A. (2003). The role of diet in cognitive decline. *Journal of neural transmission, 110*(1), 95-110.

Suo, C., Singh, M. F., Gates, N., Wen, W., Sachdev, P., Brodaty, H., . . . Singh, N. (2016). Therapeutically relevant structural and functional mechanisms triggered by physical and cognitive exercise. *Molecular psychiatry, 21*(11), 1633-1642.

Takeuchi, H., Magistro, D., Kotozaki, Y., Motoki, K., Nejad, K. K., Nouchi, R., . . . Kawashima, R. (2020). Effects of Simultaneously Performed Dual-Task Training with Aerobic Exercise and Working Memory Training on Cognitive Functions and Neural Systems in the Elderly. *Neural Plasticity, 1-17.* doi:10.1155/2020/3859824

Voss, M. W., Nagamatsu, L. S., Liu-Ambrose, T., & Kramer, A. F. (2011). Exercise, brain, and cognition across the life span. *Journal of Applied Physiology, 111*(5), 1505-1513.

Wang, H.-X., Jin, Y., Hendrie, H. C., Liang, C., Yang, L., Cheng, Y., . . . Murrell, J. R. (2013). Late life leisure activities and risk of cognitive decline. *The Journals of Gerontology Series A: Biological Sciences and Medical Sciences, 68*(2), 205-213.

Yaribeygi, H., Panahi, Y., Sahraei, H., Johnston, T. P., & Sahebkar, A. (2017). The impact of stress on body function: A review. *EXCLI journal, 16,* 1057-1072. doi:10.17179/excli2017-480

References Chapter 5

Arulsamy, A., Corrigan, F., & Collins-Praino, L. E. (2019). Cognitive and neuropsychiatric impairments vary as a function of injury severity at 12 months post-experimental diffuse traumatic brain injury: Implications for dementia development. *Behavioural Brain Research, 365,* 66-76. doi:10.1016/j. bbr.2019.02.045

Avila, J. F., Vonk, J. M. J., Verney, S. P., Witkiewitz, K., Renteria, M. A., Schupf, N., . . . Manly, J. J. (2019). Sex/gender differences in cognitive trajectories vary as a function of race/ethnicity. *Alzheimers & Dementia, 15*(12), 1516-1523. doi:10.1016/j. jalz.2019.04.006

Bennet, N. (2013). Fantasy and reality. *The Lancet, 381*(9881), 1894. doi:http://dx.doi.org/10.1016/S0140-6736(13)61147-2

Bunch, T. J., Bair, T. L., Crandall, B. G., Cutler, M. J., Day, J. D., Graves, K. G., . . . May, H. T. (2020). Stroke and dementia risk in patients with and without atrial fibrillation and carotid arterial disease. *Heart Rhythm, 17*(1), 20-26. doi:10.1016/j. hrthm.2019.07.007

Byers, A. L., Vittinghoff, E., Lui, L., Covinsky, K., Cauley, J. A., Ensrud, K., . . . Yaffe, K. (2011). CHARACTERIZATION OF LONG-TERM DEPRESSIVE TRAJECTORIES AMONG ELDERLY WOMEN. *Gerontologist, 51,* 518-518.

Cherbuin, N., Mortby, M. E., Janke, A. L., Sachdev, P. S., Abhayaratna, W. P., & Anstey, K. J. (2015). Blood Pressure, Brain Structure, and Cognition: Opposite Associations in Men and Women. *American Journal of Hypertension, 28*(2), 225-231. doi:10.1093/ajh/hpu120

Chiu, Y. L., Tsai, H. H., Lai, Y. J., Tseng, H. Y., Wu, Y. W., Peng, Y. S., . . . Chuang, Y. F. (2019). Cognitive impairment in patients with end-stage renal disease: Accelerated brain aging? *Journal of the Formosan Medical Association, 118*(5), 867-875. doi:10.1016/j.jfma.2019.01.011

Cho, Y. S., Schleifer, C., Moujaes, F., Starc, M., Ji, J. L., Santamauro, N., . . . Anticevic, A. (2018). Effects of Incentive Presentation on Spatial Working Memory Performance. *Biological Psychiatry, 83*(9), S438-S438.

Choi, S., Kim, K., Chang, J., Kim, S. M., Kim, S. J., Cho, H. J., & Park, S. M. (2019). Association of Chronic Periodontitis on Alzheimer's Disease or Vascular Dementia. *Journal of the American Geriatrics Society, 67*(6), 1234-1239. doi:10.1111/ jgs.15828 de Bruijn, R., Heeringa, J., Wolters, F. J., Franco, O. H., Stricker, B. H. C., Hofman, A., . . . Ikram, M. A. (2015). Association Between Atrial Fibrillation and Dementia in the General Population. *Jama Neurology, 72*(11), 1288-1294. doi:10.1001/jamaneurol.2015.2161

Deary, I. J., Corley, J., Gow, A. J., Harris, S. E., Houlihan, L. M., Marioni, R. E., . . . Starr, J. M. (2009). Age-associated cognitive decline. *British Medical Bulletin, 92*(1), 135-152. doi:10.1093/bmb/ldp033

Ding, J., Davis-Plourde, K. L., Sedaghat, S., Tully, P. J., Wang, W. M., Phillips, C., . . . Launer, L. J. (2020). Antihypertensive medications and risk for incident dementia and Alzheimer's disease: a meta-analysis of individual participant data from prospective cohort studies. *Lancet Neurology, 19*(1), 61-70. doi:10.1016/s1474-4422(19)30393-x

Elder, G. A., Ehrlich, M. E., & Gandy, S. (2019). Relationship of traumatic brain injury to chronic mental health problems and dementia in military veterans. *Neuroscience Letters, 707*. doi:10.1016/j.neulet.2019.134294

Fang, W. L., Jiang, M. J., Gu, B. B., Wei, Y. M., Fan, S. N., Liao, W., . . . Liu, J. (2018). Tooth loss as a risk factor for dementia: systematic review and meta-analysis of 21 observational studies. *Bmc Psychiatry, 18*. doi:10.1186/s12888-018-1927-0

Ferri, C. P., Prince, M., Brayne, C., Brodaty, H., Fratiglioni, L., Ganguli, M., . . . Alzheimers Dis, I. (2005). Global prevalence of dementia: a Delphi consensus study. *Lancet, 366*(9503), 2112-2117. doi:10.1016/s0140-6736(05)67889-0

Finsterer, J., & Stollberger, C. (2016). Neurological complications of cardiac disease (heart brain disorders). *Minerva Medica, 107*(1), 14-25.

Fletcher, J. R. Positioning ethnicity in dementia awareness research: does the use of senility risk ascribing racialised knowledge deficits to minority groups? *Sociology of Health & Illness.* doi:10.1111/1467-9566.13054

Fratiglioni, L., Mangialasche, F., & Qiu, C. (2010). Brain aging: lessons from community studies. *Nutrition Reviews, 68*(12), S119-S127. doi:10.1111/j.1753-4887.2010.00353.x

Ganguli, M., Beer, J. C., Zmuda, J. M., Ryan, C. M., Sullivan, K. J., Chang, C. C. H., & Rao, R. H. (2020). Aging, Diabetes, Obesity, and Cognitive Decline: A Population-Based Study. *Journal of the American Geriatrics Society.* doi:10.1111/jgs.16321

Gilsanz, P., Corrada, M. M., Kawas, C. H., Mayeda, E. R., Glymour, M. M., Quesenberry, C. P., . . . Whitmer, R. A. (2019). Incidence of dementia after age 90 in a multiracial cohort. *Alzheimers & Dementia, 15*(4), 497-505. doi:10.1016/j.jalz.2018.12.00

Gorelick, P. B. (2018). Prevention of cognitive impairment: scientific guidance and windows of opportunity. *Journal of Neurochemistry, 144*(5), 609-616. doi:10.1111/jnc.14113

Goulay, R., Romo, L. M., Hol, E. M., & Dijkhuizen, R. M. (2020). From Stroke to Dementia: a Comprehensive Review Exposing Tight Interactions Between Stroke and Amyloid-beta Formation. *Translational Stroke Research.* doi:10.1007/s12975-019-00755-2

Hicks, A. J., James, A. C., Spitz, G., & Ponsford, J. L. (2019). Traumatic Brain Injury as a Risk Factor for Dementia and Alzheimer Disease: Critical Review of Study Methodologies. *Journal of Neurotrauma, 36*(23), 3191-3219. doi:10.1089/neu.2018.6346

Joseph, S. J., Bhandari, S. S., & Dutta, S. (2019). Cognitive Impairment and its Correlates in Chronic Kidney Disease Patients Undergoing Haemodialysis. *Journal of Evolution of Medical and Dental Sciences-Jemds, 8*(36), 2818-2822. doi:10.14260/jemds/2019/611

Kuske, B., & Muller, S. V. (2017). First application study of he Dementia Test for People with Intellectual Disabilities (DTIM). *Zeitschrift Fur Neuropsychologie, 28*(3-4), 219-229. doi:10.1024/1016-264X/a000205

Kwon, H. S., Lee, D., Lee, M. H., Yu, S., Lim, J. S., Yu, K. H., . . . Investigators, P. (2020). Post-stroke cognitive impairment as an independent predictor of ischemic stroke recurrence: PICASSO sub-study. *Journal of Neurology.* doi:10.1007/s00415-019-09630-4

Lee, K. H., & Choi, Y. Y. (2019). Association between oral health and dementia in the elderly: a population-based study in Korea. *Scientific Reports, 9.* doi:10.1038/s41598-019-50863-0

Ma, L. Z., Huang, Y. Y., Wang, Z. T., Li, J. Q., Hou, X. H., Shen, X. N., . . . Alzheimers Dis Neuroimaging, I. (2019). Metabolically healthy obesity reduces the risk of Alzheimer's disease in elders: a longitudinal study. *Aging-Us, 11*(23), 10939-10951. doi:10.18632/aging.102496

McKenzie, K., Metcalfe, D., & Murray, G. (2018). A review of measures used in the screening, assessment and diagnosis of dementia in people with an intellectual disability. *Journal of Applied Research in Intellectual Disabilities, 31*(5), 725-742. doi:10.1111/jar.12441

Meysami, S., Raji, C. A., Merrill, D. A., Porter, V. R., & Mendez, M. F. (2019). MRI Volumetric Quantification in Persons with a History of Traumatic Brain Injury and Cognitive Impairment. *Journal of Alzheimers Disease, 72*(1), 293-300. doi:10.3233/jad-190708

Mukadam, N., Sommerlad, A., Huntley, J., & Livingston, G. (2019). Potential for dementia prevention in Latin America and Africa based on population-attributable fraction estimates. *Lancet Global Health, 7*(10), E1325-E1325. doi:10.1016/s2214-109x(19)30331-6

Mukamal, K. J., Kuller, L. H., Fitzpatrick, A. L., Longstreth, W. T., Mittleman, M. A., & Siscovick, D. S. (2003). Prospective-study of alcohol consumption and risk of dementia in older adults. *Jama-Journal of the American Medical Association, 289*(11), 1405-1413. doi:10.1001/jama.289.11.1405

Orr, M. E., Reveles, K. R., Yeh, C. K., Young, E. H., & Han, X. L. Can oral health and oral-derived biospecimens predict progression of dementia? *Oral Diseases.* doi:10.1111/odi.13201

Pazos, P., Leira, Y., Dominguez, C., Pias-Peleteiro, J. M., Blanco, J., & Aldrey, J. M. (2018). Association between periodontal disease and dementia: A literature review. *Neurologia, 33*(9), 602-613. doi:10.1016/j.nrl.2016.07.013

Petkus, A., Reynolds, C. A., Wetherell, J., Pedersen, N. L., & Gatz, M. (2015). ANXIETY, DEPRESSION AND COGNITIVE PERFORMANCE IN OLDER SWEDISH TWINS: SEX DIFFERENCES AND GENETIC INFLUENCES. *Gerontologist, 55,* 425-426.

Rahman, A., Jackson, H., Hristov, H., Isaacson, R. S., Saif, N., Shetty, T., . . . Mosconi, L. (2019). Sex and Gender Driven Modifiers of Alzheimer's: The Role for Estrogenic Control Across Age, Race, Medical, and Lifestyle Risks. Frontiers in Aging *Neuroscience, 11.* doi:10.3389/fnagi.2019.00315

Schneider, A. L. C., Selvin, E., Liang, M. L., Latour, L., Turtzo, L. C., Koton, S., . . . Gottesman, R. F. (2019). Association of Head Injury with Brain Amyloid Deposition: The ARIC-PET Study. *Journal of Neurotrauma, 36*(17), 2549-2557. doi:10.1089/neu.2018.6213

Sindi, S., Hagman, G., Hakansson, K., Kulmala, J., Nilsen, C., Kareholt, I., . . . Kivipelto, M. (2017). Midlife Work-Related Stress Increases Dementia Risk in Later Life: The CAIDE 30-Year Study. *Journals of Gerontology Series B-Psychological Sciences and Social Sciences, 72*(6), 1044-1053. doi:10.1093/geronb/gbw043

Spielberg, J. M., Sadeh, N., Leritz, E. C., McGlinchey, R. E., Milberg, W. P., Hayes, J. P., & Salat, D. H. (2017). Higher Serum Cholesterol Is Associated With Intensified Age-Related Neural Network Decoupling and Cognitive Decline in Early- to Mid-Life. *Human Brain Mapping, 38*(6), 3249-3261. doi:10.1002/hbm.23587

Tseng, L. Y., Huang, S. T., Peng, L. N., Chen, L. K., & Hsiao, F. Y. (2019). Benzodiazepines, z-Hypnotics, and Risk of Dementia: Special Considerations of Half-Lives and Concomitant Use. *Neurotherapeutics.* doi:10.1007/s13311-019-00801-9

Voros, V., Gutierrez, D. M., Alvarez, F., Boda-Jorg, A., Kovacs, A., Tenyi, T., . . . Osvath, P. (2020). The impact of depressive mood and cognitive impairment on quality of life of the elderly. *Psychogeriatrics.* doi:10.1111/psyg.12495

Walker, K. A., Sharrett, A. R., Wu, A. Z., Schneider, A. L. C., Albert, M., Lutsey, P. L., . . . Gottesman, R. F. (2019). Association of Midlife to Late-Life Blood Pressure Patterns With Incident Dementia. *Jama-Journal of the American Medical Association, 322*(6), 535-545. doi:10.1001/jama.2019.10575

Ward, A. R., & Parkes, J. (2017). An evaluation of a Singing for the Brain pilot with people with a learning disability and memory problems or a dementia. *Dementia-International Journal of Social Research and Practice, 16*(3), 360-374. doi:10.1177/1471301215592539

Wong, M. C. S., Kwan, M. W. M., Wang, H. H. X., Fong, B. C. Y., Chan, W. M., Zhang, D. X., . . . Griffiths, S. M. (2015). Dietary counselling with the Dietary Approaches to Stop Hypertension (DASH) diet for Chinese patients with grade 1 hypertension: a parallel-group, randomised controlled trial. *The Lancet, 386, Supplement 1,* S8. doi:http://dx.doi.org/10.1016/S0140-6736(15)00586-3

Yang, J. R., Kuo, C. F., Chung, T. T., & Liao, H. T. (2019). Increased Risk of Dementia in Patients with Craniofacial Trauma: A Nationwide Population-Based Cohort Study. *World Neurosurgery, 125,* E563-E574. doi:10.1016/j. wneu.2019.01.133

Yeh, Y. C., Kuo, Y. T., Huang, M. F., Hwang, S. J., Tsai, J. C., Kuo, M. C., & Chen, C. S. (2019). Association of brain white matter lesions and atrophy with cognitive function in chronic kidney disease. *International Journal of Geriatric Psychiatry, 34*(12), 1826-1832. doi:10.1002/gps.5198

Yoo, J. J., Yoon, J. H., Kang, M. J., Kim, M., & Oh, N. (2019). The effect of missing teeth on dementia in older people: a nationwide population-based cohort study in South Korea. *Bmc Oral Health, 19.* doi:10.1186/s12903-019-0750-4

Zhang, T., Li, H., Zhang, J. Y., Li, X., Qi, D., Wang, N., & Zhang, Z. J. (2016). Impacts of High Serum Total Cholesterol Level on Brain Functional Connectivity in Non-Demented Elderly. *Journal of Alzheimers Disease, 50*(2), 455-463. doi:10.3233/ jad-150810

References Chapter 6

Ajani, U. A., Ford, E. S., & Mokdad, A. H. (2004). Dietary Fiber and C-Reactive Protein: Findings from National Health and Nutrition Examination Survey Data. *Journal of Nutrition, 134*(5), 1181-1185.

Budge, M., Johnston, C., Hogervorst, E., De Jager, C., Milwain, E., Iversen, S. D., . . . Smith, A. D. (2000). Plasma total homocysteine and cognitive performance in a volunteer elderly population. In R. N. Kalaria & P. Ince (Eds.), *Vascular Factors in Alzheimer's Disease* (Vol. 903, pp. 407-410).

Butterfield, D. A., Castegna, A., Pocernich, C. B., Drake, J., Scapagnini, G., & Calabrese, V. (2002). Nutritional approaches to combat oxidative stress in Alzheimer's disease. *Journal of Nutritional Biochemistry, 13*(8), 444-461. doi:10.1016/s0955-2863(02)00205-x

Coppen, A., & Bailey, J. (2000). Enhancement of the antidepressant action of fluoxetine by folic acid: a randomised, placebo controlled trial. *Journal of Affective Disorders, 60*(2), 121-130. doi:10.1016/s0165-0327(00)00153-1

Deary, I. J., Corley, J., Gow, A. J., Harris, S. E., Houlihan, L. M., Marioni, R. E., . . . Starr, J. M. (2009). Age-associated cognitive decline. *British Medical Bulletin, 92*(1), 135-152. doi:10.1093/bmb/ldp033

Fotuhi, M., Mohassel, P., & Yaffe, K. (2009). Fish consumption, long-chain omega-3 fatty acids and risk of cognitive decline or Alzheimer disease: a complex association. *Nature Clinical Practice Neurology, 5*(3), 140-152. doi:10.1038/ncpneuro1044

Gomez-Pinilla, F. (2008). Brain foods: the effects of nutrients on brain function. *Nature Reviews Neuroscience, 9*(7), 568-578. doi:10.1038/nrn2421

Gomez-Pinilla, F. (2008). The influences of diet and exercise on mental health through hormesis. *Ageing Research Reviews,* *7*(1), 49-62. doi:10.1016/j.arr.2007.04.003

Herbison, C. E., Hickling, S., Allen, K. L., O'Sullivan, T. A., Robinson, M., Bremner, A. P., . . . Oddy, W. H. (2012). Low intake of B-vitamins is associated with poor adolescent mental health and behaviour. *Preventive Medicine*. doi:10.1016/j.ypmed.2012.09.014

Le Coutre, J., Mattson, M. P., Dillin, A., Friedman, J., & Bistrian, B. (2013). Nutrition and the biology of human ageing: Cognitive decline/food intake & caloric restriction. *Journal of Nutrition Health & Aging, 17*(8), 717-720. doi:10.1007/s12603-013-0375-2

Mathers, J. C. (2013). Nutrition and ageing: knowledge, gaps and research priorities. *Proceedings of the Nutrition Society, 72*(2), 246-250. doi:10.1017/s0029665112003023

Ordovas. (2008). *Nutrition and cognitive health*. London: The Government Office of science.

Parker, A., Fonseca, S., & Carding, S. R. (2020). Gut microbes and metabolites as modulators of blood-brain barrier integrity and brain health. *Gut Microbes, 11*(2), 135-157. doi:10.1080/19490976.2019.1638722

Pinilla, F. G. (2006). The impact of diet and exercise on brain plasticity and disease. *Nutrition and Health, 18*(3), 277-284.

Raji, C. A., Erickson, K. I., Lopez, O. L., Kuller, L. H., Gach, H. M., Thompson, P. M., . . . Becker, J. T. (2014). Regular Fish Consumption and Age-Related Brain Gray Matter Loss. *American Journal of Preventive Medicine, 47*(4), 444-451. doi:10.1016/j.amepre.2014.05.037

Sanchez-Villegas, A., Doreste, J., Schlatter, J., Rastrollo, M., & Martinez-Gonzalez, M. A. (2009). Association between folate, vitamin B-6 and vitamin B-12 intake and depression in the SUN cohort study. *Journal of Human Nutrition and Dietetics, 22*(2), 122-133. doi:10.1111/j.1365-277X.2008.00931.x

Sizonenko, S. V., Babiloni, C., Sijben, J. W., & Walhovd, K. B. (2013). Brain Imaging and Human Nutrition: Which Measures to Use in Intervention Studies? *Advances in Nutrition, 4*(5), 554-556. doi:10.3945/an.113.004283

Skarupski, K. A., Tangney, C., Li, H., Ouyang, B., Evans, D. A., & Morris, M. C. (2010). Longitudinal association of vitamin B-6, folate, and vitamin B-12 with depressive symptoms among older adults over time. *American Journal of Clinical Nutrition, 92*(2), 330-335. doi:10.3945/ajcn.2010.29413

Van Dyk, K., & Sano, M. (2007). The impact of nutrition on cognition in the elderly. *Neurochemical Research, 32*(4-5), 893-904. doi:10.1007/s11064-006-9241-5

Wärnberg, J., Gomez-Martinez, S., Romeo, J., Díaz, L. E., & Marcos, A. (2009). Nutrition, inflammation, and cognitive function *Annals of the New York Academy of Sciences* (Vol. 1153, pp. 164-175).

Witte, V. A., Kerti, L., Hermannstaedter, H. M., Fiebach, J. B., Schuchardt, J. P., Hahn, A., & Floeel, A. (2013). Effects of Omega-3 Supplementation on Brain Structure and Function in Healthy Elderly Subjects. *Journal of Psychophysiology, 27,* 45-45.

Wyatt, K. M., Dimmock, P. W., Jones, P. W., & O'Brien, P. M. S. (1999). Efficacy of vitamin B-6 in the treatment of premenstrual syndrome: systematic review. *Bmj-British Medical Journal, 318*(7195), 1375-1381. doi:10.1136/bmj.318.7195.1375

References Chapter 7

Anstey, K. J., von Sanden, C., Salim, A., & O'Kearney, R. (2007). Smoking as a risk factor for dementia and cognitive decline: a meta-analysis of prospective studies. *American journal of epidemiology, 166*(4), 367-378.

Blennow, K., de Leon, M. J., & Zetterberg, H. (2006). Alzheimer's disease. *The Lancet, 368*(9533), 387-403. doi:http://dx.doi.org/10.1016/S0140-6736(06)69113-7

Buckner, R. L. (2004). Memory and Executive Function in Aging and AD: Multiple Factors that Cause Decline and Reserve Factors that Compensate. *Neuron, 44*(1), 195-208. doi:http://dx.doi.org/10.1016/j.neuron.2004.09.006

Deal, J. A., Power, M. C., Palta, P., Alonso, A., Schneider, A. L. C., Perryman, K., . . . Sharrett, A. R. (2020). Relationship of Cigarette Smoking and Time of Quitting with Incident Dementia and Cognitive Decline. *Journal of the American Geriatrics Society, 68*(2), 337-345.

Farrow, M., Ellis, K., Matters, Y. B., & Australia, F. (2013). *Physical Activity for Brain Health and Fighting Dementia.* Retrieved from

Heyn, P., Abreu, B. C., & Ottenbacher, K. J. (2004). The effects of exercise training on elderly persons with cognitive impairment and dementia: a meta-analysis. *Archives of Physical Medicine and Rehabilitation, 85*(10), 1694-1704.

Prince, M., Albanese, E., Guerchet, M., & Prina, M. (2014). *World Alzheimer Report 2014. Dementia and risk reduction: an analysis of protective and modifiable factors.* Retrieved from London:

Additional reference Chapter 5

Marpillat NL, Macquin-Mavier I, Tropeano AI, Bachoud-Levi AC, Maison P. Antihypertensive classes, cognitive decline and incidence of dementia: a network meta-analysis. Journal of Hypertension 2013;31(6):1073-82. doi: 10.1097/HJH.0b013e3283603f53).

Solomon A, Kareholt I, Ngandu T, Wolozin B, MacDonald SWS, Winblad B, Nissinen A, Tuomilehto J, Soininen H, Kivipelto M. Serum total cholesterol, statins and cognition in non-demented elderly. Neurobiology of Aging 2009;30(6):1006-9. doi: 10.1016/j.neurobiolaging.2007.09.012.

Fratiglioni L, Mangialasche F, Qiu C. Brain aging: lessons from community studies. Nutrition Reviews 2010;68(12):S119-S27. doi: 10.1111/j.1753-4887.2010.00353.x.

Ma CR, Yin ZX, Zhu PF, Luo JS, Shi XM, Gao X.) Blood cholesterol in late-life and cognitive decline: a longitudinal study of the Chinese elderly. Molecular Neurodegeneration 2017;12. doi: 10.1186/s13024-017-0167-y.)

Gnjidic D, Naganathan V, Ben Freedman S, Beer CE, McLachlan AJ, Figtree GA, Hilmer SN. Statin Therapy and Cognition in Older People: What is the Evidence? Current Clinical Pharmacology 2015;10(3):185-93. doi: 10.2174/157488471003150820152249.

Chatterjee S, Krishnamoorthy P, Ranjan P, Roy A, Chakraborty A, Sabharwal MS, Ro R, Agarwal V, Sardar P, Danik J, et al. Statins and Cognitive Function: an Updated Review. Current Cardiology Reports 2015;17(2). doi: 10.1007/s11886-014-0559-3

Rosenblat JD, Kakar R, McIntyre RS. The Cognitive Effects of Antidepressants in Major Depressive Disorder: A Systematic Review and Meta-Analysis of Randomized Clinical Trials. International Journal of Neuropsychopharmacology 2016;19(2). doi: 10.1093/ijnp/pyv082

Shawline Publishing Group Pty Ltd

www.shawlinepublishing.com.au

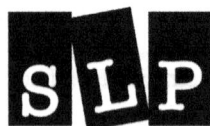

SLP

SHAWLINE
PUBLISHING
GROUP

www.ingramcontent.com/pod-product-compliance
Lightning Source LLC
Chambersburg PA
CBHW070127030426
42335CB00016B/2292